Children's surgical nursing series: 1

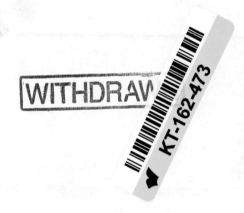

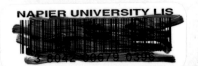

Children's surgical nursing series

Principles and practice

Children's surgical nursing series: 1

Principles and practice

by
Joanna Smith

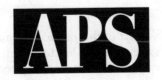

APS Publishing
The Old School, Tollard Royal, Salisbury, Wiltshire, SP5 5PW
www.apspublishing.co.uk

British Library Cataloguing in Publication Data
A catalogue record for this book is available from the British Library

© APS Publishing 2004
ISBN 1 9038770 6 7

Printed in the United Kingdom by HSW Print, Tonypandy

CONTENTS

ACKNOWLEDGEMENTS

This book is dedicated to all those working in a children's surgical environment.

I would like to express my thanks to my family and friends for their support and encouragement during the writing of this book. In particular my husband David, for his endless patience, good humour and practical help, which added to the enjoyment of writing.

I would particularly like to thank Helen Essery, Senior Sister, Children's Surgical Services, The General Infirmary at Leeds, for diligently reading and commenting on each chapter, and providing enthusiastic encouragement. I would like to thank all those who gave specialist advice including, Josie Brown (Paediatric Anaesthetist, The General Infirmary at Leeds), Maxine Robshaw (Lecturer, University of Leeds), Sharon Wood (Lecturer, University of Leeds) and Alison Twycross (Senior Lecturer, Glasgow Caledonian University).

FOREWORD

I feel very privileged to write the Foreword for this very comprehensive book and to have the opportunity of endorsing its refreshing approach and contents. To my knowledge this is a first in the UK, a text that focuses exclusively upon the issues related to children's surgical nursing, concepts and principles of care. It is truly uplifting to read a book on surgery which takes a nursing perspective and does not rely on the 'medical model' or 'systems approach' to provide the framework for the chapters.

I predict it will become a valuable companion to the myriad of books written by surgeons in the field. Within the chapters, the complexity of surgical care for children is captured. There is an appropriate balance between professional considerations and the physiological and psychological foundations of care. The anatomical and physiological distinctions between children and adults are clearly articulated and, in tune with the philosophy of children's nursing practice, there is a strong developmental theme, an emphasis on the family perspective and child's experience and, where available, strong evidence-based practice. The spotlight on spirituality is particularly refreshing.

The recently published National Service Framework recommended that all those working with children should have the appropriate knowledge and skills. This extends to those looking after children undergoing surgery in the perioperative, intra-operative and post-operative environments.

In the last decade, large strides have been made to ensure the establishment of consistent standards for children undergoing surgery. The Royal College of Surgeons—Children's Forum and the Royal College of Nursing Children's Surgical Nurses Forum have been instrumental in raising the standards for such children, and their aim is to advance the art and science of nursing in the field of children's surgery. However, many children are still looked after by staff whose knowledge and skills pertaining to children are variable. I believe that this book will appeal to children's and non-children's nurses alike, whatever their profile and learning needs, and will add to the repertoire of knowledge and skills.

Dr Annette K Dearmun
PhD BSc (Hons) RSCN RGN DN DNE RNT
Principal Lecturer—Oxford Brookes University
Senior Nurse—Oxford Radcliffe Hospital NHS Trust
Chair: Royal College of Nursing Children's Surgical Nursing Forum/Children & Young Peoples Advisory Panel

PREFACE

Children and young people require care that is appropriate and sensitive to their needs (Department of Health, 2003), delivered by a dedicated team of educated and skilled healthcare practitioners (Department of Health, 1996). Children and young people are developing individuals, with each developmental milestone having unique perspectives and challenges. Healthcare practitioners need to understand the dynamic interplay between the individual child or young person, their environment and stage of development in order to anticipate and meet their needs. The service provisions and delivery of care must not only recognise the unique needs of this important group as a whole, but also each child and young person's individuality and their family's role and contribution to care.

The current technological revolution, advances in medical treatments and increased consumerism all have a significant impact upon the health care delivery within developed societies. The increase in children's surgical specialties can be directly attributed to advances in paediatric anaesthesia and paediatric diagnostic technology, and an increased understanding of paediatric pathophysiology (Noble *et al*, 1997). As services evolve and more conditions are amenable to complex surgical treatment, new ethical and moral challenges emerge. However, working with the child and family, where the child requires surgery, provides everyday challenges for healthcare professionals, such as ensuring:

- Sensitive and appropriate preparation of a young child for surgery, where in the absence of an acute illness, he/she may not understand the need for surgery

- Swift and efficient management of the child admitted acutely for life-saving surgery, where time may be at a premium, is balanced with appropriate explanations and involving the child and family in his/her care

- The child who requires a series of procedures, which may continue through out his/her life, is involved in the decision-making process and his/her overall welfare remains paramount. Negative experiences will influence future decision-making processes.

Furthermore, as the boundaries between professionals caring for children become increasingly blurred, teamwork and an interdisciplinary approach to care are essential. The common goal is to provide high quality care, which meets the needs of the child and young person, and their families or carers. In order to meet these challenges and respond to a wide age range of children, practitioners are not only required to maintain existing skills and knowledge through basic training and education, but develop new clinical skills and new ways of working. This includes being highly knowledgeable in the physiological and psychological variables unique to children (Noble *et al*, 1997) and applying this knowledge when assessing each child's needs, planning care, instigating treatments, maintaining homeostasis, giving medication and considering the potential long-term consequences of treatment.

The aims of this series of books relating to children's surgical nursing are to provide an overview of the general principles of caring for a child requiring surgery, such as family-centred care, pain management, consent and perioperative care, and to provide the reader with detailed information for individual groups of conditions and their management, which requires predominantly surgical treatment, such as cardio-thoracic surgery, neurosurgery and gastrointestinal surgery. These aims will be achieved by dividing the subjects into texts of manageable sizes. This first text will focus upon issues relevant to all nurses working in a children's surgical setting, with subsequent complementary texts focusing on a particular specialty. Although the series is primarily aimed at nurses, both pre-registration students and qualified nurses new to a children's surgical environment, it is hoped that the series will be a valuable resource to a range of healthcare professionals, both junior and experienced, working with children and young people requiring surgery. Furthermore, it is hoped this first book will be of value to staff working in a theatre environment wishing to update and improve their knowledge of general issues relating to the care of children. Although *Chapter 4* focuses on perioperative care, it only provides an overview of the child in theatre and therefore will not provide sufficient depth for staff working predominantly within a theatre environment.

The term 'child' will be used to represent infants, children and young people, unless specific considerations require highlighting. Policy documents cited within the text are primarily from relevant health and welfare government departments in England. Many of the principles are contained within equivalent documents for Scotland, Wales and Northern Ireland. It is not within the context of this text to evaluate and include policy from an international perspective. However, it is hoped that by highlighting policy issues readers will consider how the needs of the child requiring surgery are being addressed in their own practice area, and will seek to identify appropriate guidance from within their own country. Where available, evidence-based care will be reflected upon and supported by appropriate references. In the absence of available literature to support care, descriptions will be provided based upon 'best' practice, with rationale, and an indication that there is a lack of a current evidence-base.

References

Department of Health (2003) *Getting the Right Start: National Service Framework for Children. Emerging Findings.* HMSO, London

Department of Health (1996) *National Health Service Patient's Charter: Services for Children and Young People.* HMSO, London

Noble RR, Micheli AJ, Hensley MA *et al* (1997) Perioperative considerations for the pediatric patient: a developmental approach. *Nurs Clin N Am* 23(1): 1–16

ONE

THE DEVELOPMENT OF HEALTH SERVICES FOR CHILDREN

There are approximately 12 million children in the United Kingdom, equating to approximately 20 percent of the population (Department of Health, 2003), of which it has been estimated that 25 percent of two year olds will have been a hospital inpatient and one in four children will have attended accident and emergency (House of Commons, 1997). Despite this high utilisation of services, the health expenditure (excluding births) for children is only 12 percent and includes both hospital and community care (Department of Health, 1999). Children's services are often marginalised and subsequently struggle to gain appropriate recognition, both in terms of resources and in the implementation of strategies that are necessary to ensure services meet the needs of this vulnerable group of clients (Department of Health, 2001). Services remain patchy and variable; recommendations for good practice are frequently based upon rhetoric and often have little impact upon service delivery. The first section of this chapter will provide an outline of the major reports relating to the care of children within England, highlighting areas where standards have been raised and services have evolved, while identifying recommendations for future service delivery. The second section will continue this theme, but more specifically in relation to the child requiring surgery. Finally, the drive and rationale for promoting evidence-based, and ensuring quality, care will be outlined.

1.1 Overview of current reports relating to the provision of hospital services for children

The Curtis Report (Ministry of Health, 1946) was the first report relating directly to childcare provision in the United Kingdom. Although the main remit of the Committee was to focus upon the provisions for children requiring indefinite residential care, they did consider the temporary long-term care of children in hospital. There were many aspects of the report which would now be deemed offensive, particularly in the terminology used to describe children and the number and variability of establishments in which children were living—being cared for was a rather over-optimistic statement. The Report, however, was emotive and stirred public conscience relating to the plight of many children in Britain. In general, 'sick wards' made few provisions for children in areas such as play, recreation and education, and there were inadequacies in relation to the environment, the number and suitability of staff 'caring' for the children, and parental access. This was in part due to lack of recognition that staff qualified in child care were necessary, therefore training was not generally available. Recommendations included areas in which children are cared for must be separate from adult facilities, and carers should have adequate training.

Although there had been previous studies and circulars relating to child welfare, *The Welfare of Children in Hospital*, more commonly referred to as the Platt Report (Ministry of Health, 1959), was the first to focus solely on the overall well-being of children in hospital. The Report's aim was 'to make a special study of the arrangements made in hospitals for the welfare of ill children—as distinct from their medical and nursing treatment—and to make suggestions which could be passed on to hospital care authorities' (Ministry of Health, 1959: 1). The Platt Report has been heralded as one of the most important and influential documents of its time. It was prompted by the increased awareness of children's needs, widening access to hospital treatment and increased technology. Children admitted to hospital were no longer solely from those living in poverty. At the time of the Report's commission, statistics relating to children in hospital were not generally separated from adults. There was very little information relating to the number of children requiring hospital treatment and the length of stay, let alone the experiences of the children and their families.

The central themes the Committee considered included the emotional needs of the child in hospital, the role of parents whose child is admitted to hospital, and the distress children experience when separated from their family. Topics such as education, play facilities, safety, personal possessions, food, toileting and spiritual needs were discussed. The recommendations contained within the Platt Report pivoted around the premise that every effort should be made to minimise the distress children experience in hospital as a result of separation from family and a familiar environment. Even today, this principle remains a core feature of child health care. The recommendations included:

- Staff caring for children should not only have knowledge about the specific diseases of childhood, but also factors which influence the development of the healthy child and the role of the family

- Admission to hospital wherever possible should be avoided

- The development of home care, outpatients and day care should be encouraged

- Children should not be nursed with adults

- Environment and ward designs should reflect the needs of the child

- Children should be prepared for hospital admission at the level of their understanding

- Parents should be supported in providing care for their child.

Twenty-five years after the Platt Report, the second major review of health services for children was conducted, culminating in the Court Report (*Fit for the Future; The Report of the*

Committee on Child Health Services) (Department of Health, 1976). The aim of this Report was to review existing health services for children. The findings indicated that, although there had been some service developments, there was still 'a make do and mend' situation; only 43 percent of sisters working in children's wards were Registered Sick Children's Nurses (RSCN) and the special needs of the child were not always considered (Department of Health, 1976: 8). Recommendations included:

- Services for children should be family-centred
- Services should be integrated in that there should be a comprehensive primary care focus supported by consultant and hospital care
- There should be a programme of health surveillance for all children, with additional support for children in need
- Schools should have designated nurse contact time.

The recommendations had similar philosophical underpinnings to the Platt Report, but there were more explicit recommendations in relation to child health surveillance.

In 1991, the guidance report, *Welfare of Children and Young People in Hospital* (Department of Health, 1991) was published, which aimed 'to convey results of research, writing and teaching, and the deliberations of expert bodies, to reflect the quality of widely qualified best practice given to children and their families' (p1). The Report was based on several cardinal principles that were deemed necessary to ensure that services for children provided for both their physical and emotional needs. These principles were:

- Children should only be admitted to hospital if the care they require cannot be as well provided for at home, in a day clinic or on a day basis
- Children should be discharged home as soon as possible, with appropriate support
- Involving parents/carers with care is paramount

- Facilities should be distinct and separate from adult services, with suitable accommodation for children and parents

- Children have a right to privacy and respect, to be treated with tact and understanding, and have information appropriate to their age.

These principles were translated into detailed guidance for specific settings or groups of children. Within the hospital setting, the guidance clearly states that it is desirable for children to be cared for within a children's department (or children's hospital), which should include a lead children's physician, specialist nursing services managed by a children's nurse, child-centred routines, and have play and education facilities. Staff training and education were deemed paramount, with recommendations that there should be a minimum of two RSCN/child branch nurses on duty 24 hours a day in each children's ward or department, although this number should be commensurate with children's needs. Where there is a need to utilise joint facilities with adult services, such as accident and emergency, there should be separate treatment and waiting areas. These areas should have child-specific procedures and policies, equipment appropriate to the needs of children and an RSCN/child branch nurse available for advice 24 hours a day. Children admitted to hospital should have a named paediatric consultant who has responsibility for their care, or advising upon their care if specialist care delivered by a primarily adult-focused consultant is required.

The *Welfare of Children and Young People in Hospital* (Department of Health, 1991) guidance is the current benchmark against which hospital child health services within the United Kingdom are measured. Certainly the principles within the report were embodied within the *Patients' Charter Services for Children and Young People* (Department of Health, 1996). Furthermore, the *Clothier Report* (Department of Health, 1994) (the inquiry relating to the deaths and injuries of children during the period of February to April 1991 at Grantham and Kesteven General Hospital) vehemently recommended that the Department of Health should take steps to ensure that the guidance was followed more closely. The 1993 audit of children services, *Children First; A Study of Hospital Services* (Audit Commission, 1993) examined how the principles recommended in reports relating to the child in hospital in the preceding 30 years were being upheld. The six principles which formed the structure of the report were primarily drawn from the *Welfare of Children and Young People in Hospital* (Department of Health, 1991) and centred around the following themes:

- Child and family-centred care
- Specially skilled staff
- Separate facilities
- Effective treatments
- Appropriate hospitalisation
- Strategic commissioning.

The Audit Commission's findings indicated that, although there were good examples of developments within all of the themes, these developments were patchy and overall there was poor implementation of previous guidance papers. These inadequacies included:

- Failure and inconsistencies in the implementation of family-centred care
- Inadequate facilities for parents
- Lack of appropriate junior staff able to deal with paediatric emergencies
- Lack of surgeons and anaesthetists with appropriate skills in dealing with children due to the occasional nature of their paediatric practice
- Children requiring specialist care not being referred to appropriate regional centres
- Many wards caring for children not meeting the standard of two children's trained nurses on duty each shift
- Children nursed on adult wards

- The specific needs of adolescents often not considered
- Inappropriate admission to hospital
- Lack of monitoring of the effectiveness of treatments
- Lack of clear strategies for children's services.

The most recent review of hospital services in the United Kingdom for children and young people occurred between 1996 and 1997 and was undertaken by the House of Commons Health Select Committee (House of Commons, 1997). Again there were endorsements of the principles contained within the *Welfare of Children and Young People in Hospital* guidance (Department of Health, 1991). However, there were concerns that these principles had become 'aspirations rather than actual achievements' (p.viii) and that lack of progress was a direct result of fragmentation of the services providing care for children (such as between hospital and community services, social services and education), insufficient attention or a low priority given to the provision of services for children, services not always provided by the most appropriately educated and experienced staff, and services not always designed to meet the specific health needs of children.

Reinforcement of the fragmentation of children's services and lack of national priorities for children's health care were again a strong theme within the protracted and lengthy Bristol Royal Infirmary inquiry, which investigated the poor outcomes and organisation of care for children requiring cardiac surgery, when compared with equivalent centres (Bristol Royal Infirmary, 2001). The Report recommended the need for a national director for children's services and, despite being long overdue, welcomed the government's commitment to a National Service Framework for Children.

The emerging findings of the *National Service Framework for Children: Getting the Right Start* (Department of Health, 2003) is the beginning of a vision for improving the lives and health of children through the development of effective, evidence-based and needs-led services. The document sets the scene and provides an underpinning philosophy for the future welfare of children. It contains a potential blueprint for the final framework and gives services providers direction, so that they can begin working towards local implementation. The Report has three broad aims: improving services, tackling health inequalities, and enhancing partnership between the agencies responsible for the welfare of children. The taskforce responsible for the development of the National Service Framework for Children in conjunction with the external working groups is continuing to prepare the detailed service provisions recommendations for specific groups of children. In light of the Bristol Royal Infirmary (2001) Report, the standards for the care of children in hospital have been developed first. However, the taskforce is clear that this is not a suggestion that acute care has the dominant role to play in the overall welfare of children.

The National Service Framework's standards for hospital services for children (Department of Health, 2003a) build upon the core and fundamental principles within the broader framework. The specific aim is to guide hospital services in ensuring care is delivered in a way that meets the needs of the child and family, is safe and effective and provided by appropriately trained staff. Although the principles within previous reports relating to hospital services for children have been retained, there is greater emphasis upon:

- Integration of services and fostering links with appropriate agencies that have an impact upon the child's welfare

- The overall experiences of the child and family

- Ensuring children and their families work in partnership with hospitals in the development of services

- Clinical governance and the quality agenda being central to service provision

- Improved education and training of all staff caring for children

- Environmental and safety issues.

Despite the wealth of advice and guidance papers relating to provision of health services for children within the National Health Service, to date there has been a recurrent failure to make significant inroads in implementing these recommendations. The National Service Framework programme, as a government initiative (Department of Health, 1998; Department of Health, 1997), probably offers the greatest potential at present for ensuring that appropriate healthcare provisions for children are secured. All healthcare professionals working with children need to contribute to the process and continue to pressurise government, health authorities and local services providers into ensuring recommendations are followed. Unfortunately, there are many reasons why the key principles relating to meeting the health needs of children are not met, including the difficulties in effecting change through national guidance papers. Services are often based on rituals and traditions rather than the needs of the children, and there is a lack of suitably qualified staff.

There are no easy solutions to these dilemmas. However, possible strategies, as recommended by the Select Committee (House of Commons, 1997), include:

- Developing community children's nursing in areas where there are shortfalls, which should be integrated with other children's services

- Ensuring accurate information is collected in relation to the number of children (and adolescents) admitted to hospital, where children are cared for, and under which specialty

- Developing and introducing performance-monitoring tools

- Addressing training issues, particularly the shortfall in children's nurses

- Identifying a lead commissioner for child health services within each commissioning authority

- Encouraging local solutions to meet local needs, in particular in collaborative working and sharing ideas.

1.2   Children's surgery in context

Technological advances in surgical and anaesthetic techniques have resulted in more children with complex disorders being treated. These advances, combined with changing attitudes towards the care of children, have resulted in the development of children's surgery becoming a specialist field in its own right (Heath, 1998).

The first recorded anaesthetic to be administered to a child was in 1842 (Burns, 1997). Although there had been reports of surgical treatments for children much earlier (Touloukian, 1995), this led to pioneering work in the field of children's surgery by Dennis-Brown in the United Kingdom, and Hirschsprung and later Lladd in the United States of America (Noble *et al*, 1997; Touloukian, 1995). Their contribution has left a legacy for present day paediatric surgical practice, including:

- The recognition that child's anatomy and physiology are different from those of an adult

- The need for proper diagnosis, skilled anaesthetists and appropriate peri-operative care for the child and family.

(Burns, 1997; Noble *et al*, 1997; Touloukian, 1995)

Despite these early and promising beginnings, the specific needs of children requiring surgery, in common with children's services, have in general been of low priority in an increasingly stretched health service. The Department of Health (1993) Audit Commission report identified that 44 percent of children admitted to hospital require a surgical procedure (*figure 1.2a*), of which two thirds are elective admissions. This was probably the first time that the major contribution surgical specialities make to the healthcare of children was highlighted. The Audit Commission found that many previous reports and guidance papers relating to the care of children in hospital were not being considered and that this was most striking within the area of surgery. Most obvious was the continued practice of admitting children requiring surgery to adult surgical wards, with surgeons preferring this option on the basis that nurses required disease-specific knowledge rather than specialist knowledge of children. This has often resulted in there being little regard to the overall welfare and emotional well-being of the child, or understanding of the needs of the family. The Audit Commission (1993) questioned the ability of medical staff to maintain and develop their skills in paediatric care in light of the fact that many surgeons and anaesthetists had only occasional paediatric practice.

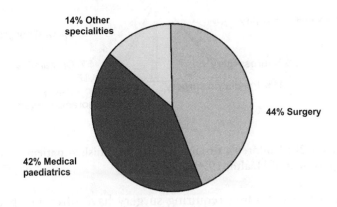

14% Other specialities

44% Surgery

42% Medical paediatrics

Figure 1.2a: Paediatric admissions to hospital (Audit Commission, 1993)

The most recent figures relating to children's surgical admissions divided into specialities were published in 1999 (Department of Health, 1999a). The only real changes in surgical admissions in terms of specialities since 1993 occurred in the field of general surgery, where there has been a reduction in children admitted under the care of adult general surgeons from 32 percent to 15 percent. However, this is counterbalanced by an increased workload in paediatric surgeons from 6.8 percent to 11 percent, with a further 3 percent of children managed by paediatric urologists, now a recognised sub-division within paediatric surgery. Ear, nose and throat surgery is the most common reason children are admitted to hospital (Audit Commission,

1993) and accounts for 29 percent of the total paediatric surgical workload (Department of Health, 1999a). The breakdown of surgery into specialisms is represented in *Figure 1.2b*.

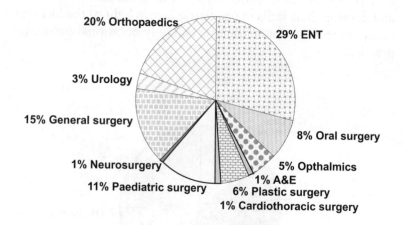

Figure 1.2b: Children's surgical admission, finished patient episodes (Department of Health, 1999)

The reasons children requiring surgery have often not been a high priority include:

- Rigid organisational structures

- Children's surgical wards not always managed within children's service directorates

- Lack of children's nurses holding senior positions within organisations

- Barriers imposed by surgical and anaesthetic colleagues whose main workload and priorities may lie with adult services

- Lack of knowledge or unable to implement guidance reports relating to the welfare of children in hospital.

Issues that have concerned nurses (and perhaps still do) include:

- Excessive and rigid fasting of children due to the imposition of standard adult-focused policies
- Lack of multidisciplinary pain management guidelines specific for children
- Parents unable to have the choice of escorting their child to the anaesthetic room or be with their child in recovery
- Rigid ward routines
- Lack of adolescent facilities
- Lack of community care upon discharge.

The utilisation of guidance paper can provide leverage to improve services for children requiring surgery. *Getting the Right Start: National Service Framework for Children. Standards for Hospital Services* (Department of Health, 2003a) (sections 4.34–4.39) outlines the specific service provision for children requiring surgery. However, the two main documents that have explicit standards for the nursing care of children requiring surgery are *Just for the Day* (Thornes, 1991) and *Setting Standards for Children Undergoing Surgery* (Hogg, 1994). Although both probably require updating, they still offer the best available guidance for nurses caring for children undergoing surgery. The principles contained within *Just for the Day* will be discussed in depth in *Chapter 7*.

Setting Standards for Children Undergoing Surgery was published in an attempt to address many of the inadequacies and concerns that nurses caring for children undergoing surgery face within everyday practice. The standards are formulated into key statements with criteria on how to meet these statements, for both healthcare professionals and commissioners of services:

- The decision to operate
- Admission to hospital
- Preparation for operation
- Ward procedures
- Going to theatre

- Anaesthetic room
- Recovery room
- After the operation
- Home again.

The standards are an excellent starting point for all staff involved in the care of children undergoing surgery. The easy-to-use checklist enables the user to identify both standards which require improving upon, and those which are non-existent and therefore require developing. The standards could easily be adapted into a benchmarking framework (discussed in *Section 1.3*). The overall standards appear to be based upon sound principles. However, in today's evidence-based climate, nurses wishing to fully utilise the standards will need to conduct and critique more current literature to supplement the standards and bring them up-to-date.

Although not specifically aimed at nursing staff, there are several key documents which have the potential to radically alter the management of the care of children undergoing surgery in the United Kingdom; for example, *Children's Surgical Services* (Royal College of Paediatrics and Child Health, 1996), *Extremes of Age* (Royal College of Anaesthetists, 1999) and *Children's Surgery—A First Class Service* (Paediatric Forum of the Royal College of Surgeons, 2000). Certainly nurses could and should be using the principles within these documents to consider new ways of working. The key points from *Children's Surgery—A First Class Service* are important because of their potential to shape the organisation of future services for children admitted to hospital for primarily surgical treatment.

The Report, along with the establishment of a paediatric forum within the Royal College of Surgeons, is a clear commitment by the College that it recognises children as having different needs from adults and as such cannot be treated as small adults. Embodied within the Report is the emphasis that *all* children undergoing surgery receive the highest possible standards of care appropriate to their needs, while ensuring maximum safety. The aims included:

- Defining national standards for the management of children requiring surgery
- Ensuring children receive treatment in an appropriate environment
- Ensuring adequate training, education and assessment for surgeons involved in the care of children
- Promoting audit and quality initiatives.

In order to address these aims, the specific recommendations included:

- Occasional paediatric practice is unacceptable. However, this must be counterbalanced with the need to provide local surgical services for children, in order to minimise the disruption that can result from travelling to geographically distant centres
- Inpatient surgery should only be performed at hospitals that provide comprehensive paediatric facilities
- Only appropriately trained and designated surgeons, whose paediatric workload is of sufficient volume to maintain competence, should carry out surgery on children
- Specialist centres should be more integrated and work in collaboration with district general hospitals
- The clinical management structure should involve a multidisciplinary group representing surgeons, anaesthetists, paediatricians and children's nurses.

The document was clear in its belief that the care of children should be under the direction of nurses specifically educated in the care of sick children. Many children's nurses will undoubtedly welcome these recommendations and use this document as an opportunity to work in collaboration with surgical and anaesthetic colleagues, in order to ensure the child admitted for a surgical procedure not only has the best available surgery, but their health needs are addressed in an holistic manner.

1.3: The provision of quality care

In the United Kingdom, the increased focus upon evidence-based practice during the 1990s is in part due to the greater importance government policy has placed upon the need to enhance the quality of care and clinical effectiveness within the National Health Service (Department of Health, 1998; National Health ServiceExecutive, 1998; 1996), the overall aim being to reduce variations in clinical practice and improve standards of care for all patients. Clinical effectiveness had been defined as the extent which clinical interventions (for a particular patient or population) do what they are intended to do, which is to maintain and improve health (National Health Service Executive, 1996). Some of the benefits of delivering clinically-effective care are as follows:

- Reduced time wasted on inappropriate treatments
- Reduced variations of services and increased consistency of care
- Increased patient understanding of investigations and treatments
- Increased patient confidence in healthcare professionals and the National Health Service
- Increased value for money and promoting cost effectiveness
- Using clinical audit to enhance the quality of care.

(le May, 2000)

In order to ensure a quality service, healthcare professionals must ensure care is clinically effective. This can be achieved by redefining and changing practice in accordance with current evidence, and integrating activities such as research, clinical audit, and continued professional development into the clinical workplace. The Department of Health document, *A First Class Service: Quality in the National Health Service (Department of Health, 1998) outlines* clinical governance as the framework through which the National Health Service will achieve clinical effectiveness. McSherry and Haddock (1999) describe clinical governance as an umbrella term, which brings together key themes that are central to the quality assurance process, namely:

- Healthcare professionals having the correct skills, knowledge and competencies to undertake their role efficiently and effectively

- Ensuring practice is based upon the most recent evidence by accessing, implementing, monitoring, supervising and disseminating research findings

- Undertaking clinical risk analysis and audit to ensure efficient and effective standards of care are developed and maintained.

Delivering high quality patient care within the clinical governance framework requires more than establishing systems to coordinate the process of quality assurance (Royal College of Nursing, 2000). There must be a concurrent fundamental change in culture that promotes and supports improvements in clinical practice. This includes having clear lines of responsibility and accountability, openness, sharing information and developing partnerships between professionals, and supporting continued professional development. A critical component within the quality framework is the need to identify and build upon good practice, with evidence-based practice spearheading the process.

The evidence-based practice movement within the health arena has, to date, been led by the medical profession. Thus it is hardly surprising that Sackett *et al*'s (1996) definition of evidence-based medicine, 'the conscientious, explicit and judicious use of current best evidence in making clinical decisions about the care of individual patients', is the most widely adopted (p71). Muir Gray (2001) offered a broader definition stating that evidence-based clinical practice is 'an approach to decision-making, in which the clinician uses the best evidence available, in consultation with the patient, to decide upon the option which suits the patient best' (p17). Within nursing, these definitions may not be appropriate because of the orientation towards randomised clinical trials as the 'gold standard' for evidence and the need for nurses to incorporate tacit knowledge into the decision-making process (French, 1999: 74). French offers an alternative definition of evidence-based practice, which is 'the systematic interconnecting of scientifically generated evidence with the tacit knowledge of the expert practitioner to achieve a change in a particular practice for the benefit of a well-defined client/patient group'. The drawback of this definition is the lack of consideration for the individual client and their contribution to the decision-making process. The advantage is the implicit focus on the practitioners' experiences, which, integrated with current research, is a real way of reducing the so-called theory/practice gap.

Flemming (1998), based upon Sackett *et al*'s (1997) work, has suggested a five-stage process, which nurses can use as a framework, in order to develop their practice based upon evidence:

- Identification of structured questions, derived from practice situations

- Identification of external evidence from research by undertaking a literature review

- Critical appraisal of the research in terms of validity and reliability

- Utilisation of the best available evidence, alongside clinical expertise and the patient's perspective, to deliver care

- Evaluation of performance through self-reflection, audit or peer assessment.

Certainly nurses need to be able to identify aspects of practice that have uncertainties and from these, clarify the actual issue/s that require addressing. The next stage would be to undertake a comprehensive literature review and evaluate the available evidence. Muir Gray (2001: 104) suggests that evidence can be categorised into five areas, ranked in order of strength:

Type 1: evidence in the form of a systematic review of multiple well-designed randomised control trials

Type 2: evidence from at least one properly designed random-
         ised control trial of an appropriate size

Type 3: evidence from well-designed trials without random-
         isation, single group pre-post, cohort, time series or
         matched case-control studies

Type 4: evidence from well-designed non-experimental studies
         from more than one centre or research group

Type 5: opinions of respected authorities based on clinical evi-
         dence, descriptive studies or reports of external com-
         mittees.

This ranking supports the quantitative paradigm. Clarke (1999)
argues that, although evidence in the form of research is vital in
its contribution to the decision-making process, it could also be
a retrograde step to ignore the humanistic and personal experiences that contribute to delivering quality care. Best evidence is
the evidence that helps the client most, and it cannot be assumed
that this will always be in the form of quantitative research, as
exemplified by the randomised control trial (Clarke, 1999). Not
all nursing literature supports this view; DiCenso and Cullum
(1998) suggest that the randomised control trial is the most
effective design for evaluating a nursing intervention than other
categories of evidence, with qualitative studies offering a
method for understanding the attitudes and beliefs of patients.
Cheater and Closs (1997) suggest that evidence generated from
qualitative research is essential if clinical problems are to be
understood and are particularly relevant if little is known about
a topic, allowing a hypothesis to be generated and tested. The
value of the qualitative approach would seem particularly pertinent within nursing when the research base is at the beginning of
its development. What constitutes best evidence very much
depends upon the clinical question that requires addressing and
the type and quality of evidence research available. This position
does not endorse either the qualitative or quantitative paradigm.

   Obtaining relevant evidence is just the start of the process.
The evidence has to be critically appraised and utilised in the
practice setting. The publication of *Getting Evidence into Practice* (Effective Health Care Bulletin, 1999) clearly indicates that

quality care can only be achieved by shifting the emphasis from research generation to the implementation of evidence into practice. The National Health Service Executive (1996; 1998) and Department of Health (1995) have suggested several approaches to getting evidence into practice, including:

- Clinical guidelines and protocols
- Standard setting and benchmarking
- Education materials (conferences, lectures, seminars, learning sets)
- Decision support systems
- Opinion leaders
- Clinical audit
- Market research strategies.

Guidelines and benchmarking will be explored in more detail because of their increasing popularity within clinical practice. The use of research-based clinical guidelines have been identified as an ideal way of getting evidence into practice (McClarey, 1998). Field and Lohr (1992) assert that guidelines are systematically developed statements, which assist the practitioner to make clinical decisions, with the patient, about the appropriate health care delivery, for a specific clinical circumstance. Grimshaw and Russell (1994) suggest that guidelines should include explicit recommendations for clinical practice based upon scientific evidence. Woolf *et al* (1999) summarised the potential advantages and disadvantages of clinical guidelines; advantages are summarised as:

- Promoting care which has proven benefit and discouraging care which is not based on evidence
- Improving the consistency of care
- Information can be summarised or adapted into patients' information leaflets
- Influencing policy

- Easily accessible with explicit information for healthcare professionals
- The first stage in developing quality assessment tools
- Cost effective
- Improving efficiency.

Disadvantages would be:

- The guideline may not represent current best evidence or the views of a misrepresented minority
- Cost may have taken precedent over patient needs
- Inflexible
- Do not respond to individual needs.

The use of clinical guidelines can be problematic, particularly translating research findings and transferring information into everyday practice (Hopkins, 1995:72). Hopkins states that 'the core feature of clinical guidelines is that they should be based upon good scientific evidence'. This, however, creates a problem when there is a paucity of high quality research.

Associated developmental strategies are necessary if guidelines (and, in fact, other approaches of getting evidence in to practice) are to be effective and change practice. A systematic review of implementing clinical guidelines (Effective Health Care Bulletin, 1994) suggests that guidelines are more likely to be successfully implemented if they reflect local needs. The practical issues, which require addressing in order to develop and implement clinical guidelines, include: who should develop the guidelines, how the guidelines should be developed, and dissemination and implementation of the guidelines. Developing strategies to implement and disseminate guidelines is crucial if a change in practice is to take place. Thomas *et al* (1999) indicate that active dissemination strategies (through educational packages, lecturers and training sessions, restructuring documentation) are more likely to bring about a change in practice when compared to more passive dissemination strategies (such as journal publications).

If the quality of care is to be improved, then a system needs to develop whereby current practice can be compared with practice standards and an action plan developed to remedy any deficiencies (Crombie *et al*, 1993). Evaluation of care is central to the quality process; therefore it is not surprising that clinical audit is a prominent feature within the quality agenda. Dixon (1991) defines audit as 'the systematic peer evaluation of the quality of patient care, based on explicit and measurable indicators of quality, for the purpose of demonstrating and improving the quality of patient care' (p28). The purpose of audit is to review the delivery of care in order to identify areas where improvements can be made (Harvey, 1995). Thus, the development of guidelines should be linked to the audit process. However, it is neither desirable nor possible to collect data on all aspects of care contained within a guideline (Crombie *et al*, 1993). Standards or criteria need to be formulated from the guidelines with these becoming elements subsequently audited. The success of the audit process requires teamwork, designated time to develop, implementing and reviewing the standards, and education of all staff in relation to the outcomes and changes needed to improve practice (Harvey, 1995). It is an ongoing cyclical process.

The New NHS: Modern and Dependable (Department of Health, 1997: 33) clearly identifies that it is the responsibility of every healthcare practitioner to ensure that every patient receives quality care. In addition, the variability and inconsistencies in care across services must be reduced and there must be a sharing of best practice. Clinical benchmarking has become a popular framework for seeking, finding, implementing and sustaining best practice. Benchmarking has the potential to improve standards of care and can be a means of developing best practice, where the benchmark acts as the standard against which services and practices can be compared (Ellis and Morris, 1997). *Figure 1.3a* represent the cyclical process of benchmarking. The *NHS Plan* (Department of Health, 2000) reinforced the need to improve the overall patient experience, starting with getting the basics right. The *Essence of Care* (Department of Health, 2001a) toolkit was designed to support the quality agenda by setting out national clinical benchmarks in eight key care areas: self-care, hygiene, nutrition, continence, pressure ulcers, safety in mental health, record-keeping, and privacy and dignity. The clinical benchmarks not only include the best available evidence to support practice, but were developed with patients and carers. Chambers and Jolly (2002) suggest the national toolkit is already having an impact, for example:

- Direct patient care, particularly in relation to improving nutrition provision and improving patient education
- Influencing strategic decision-making, i.e. by incorporating the benchmarks into clinical governance agendas
- Influencing service developments, i.e. by basing models of care on the benchmarks
- Integrating the benchmarks into education programmes.

However, implementing the *Essence of Care* (Department of Health, 2001a) toolkit is not without challenges (Chambers and Jolly, 2002), and these include:

- Lack of dedicated funding for implementation
- Shifting responsibility of quality to the individual, which may cause additional stresses to an already stretched workforce
- Turning enthusiasm into sustainable commitment
- The limited range of clinical benchmarks currently available.

In addition, within the child health setting, the benchmarks may be viewed as having been developed primarily for adult patients (Jones, 2003). Certainly this is reflected in adult bias in relation to the range of supporting evidence and lack of indication as to the involvement of parents and children as a distinct user group. Furthermore, national benchmarks do not consider the context of care and the actual needs of the clients, which may be very varied (Ellis, 2000).

Benchmarking has been well established within the child health arena, with the formulation in 1994 of the North West Paediatric Benchmarking Group (Ellis, 1995). Through the

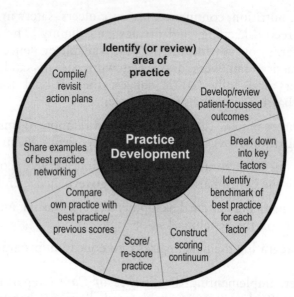

Figure1.3a: Benchmarking framework (adapted from Ellis *et al*, 2000)

work of benchmarking groups, practitioners are able to share practice, discuss areas of concern, provide practical support and encouragement and, most importantly, minimise duplication of effort thereby encouraging efficient use of resources (Ellis and Morris, 1997). Ellis (2000; 1995) suggests that benchmarking has advantages over other types of quality initiatives including:

- Practitioners lead the quality process, therefore clinical needs are addressed and benchmarks are developed that are realistic

- Practitioners value the process and the process values practitioners and recognises individual efforts

- Benchmarks are not dependent upon the existence of high quality research; a range of evidence including professional consensus is utilised

- Benchmarks represent the best possible care for the patient

- Benchmarks are measurable

- Benchmarks are audited locally and can be compared with other areas
- Action plans ensure change is encouraged and therefore practice develops
- Revisiting areas of practice ensures benchmarks are updated and scoring is a cyclical process
- There is effective sharing of resources.

As with guidelines, benchmarking has drawbacks. Although one of the strengths of clinical benchmarking is that all evidence is viewed for its own worth and not ranked in a hierarchical system (Ellis, 2000), there is a potential for benchmarks not to represent current best evidence, but instead come to symbolise the views of a misrepresented minority. Furthermore, membership of the group must vary to ensure that professionals with the relevant expertise and knowledge are actively encouraged to contribute or again there is a danger that the benchmark will not represent current best practice. The North West Paediatric Benchmarking Group has, to date, excluded the child and family from contributing to the process of developing benchmarks (Ellis, 2000), and perhaps this is a challenge for the future. In order for benchmarking to be successful, it is dependent upon practitioners' willingness to share, honesty when scoring benchmarks and openness when comparing results (Ellis, 2000;1995).

Identifying sources of evidence can be problematic and currently nursing has many areas of practice which simply do not have an evidence base (English and Bond, 1998; Smith and Callaghan, 2001). There is a danger that the lack of evidence base within nursing has the potential to stifle the development of guidelines and reduce the robustness of the benchmarking process. The paucity of credible published studies is a particular concern, together with the lack of involvement of children within the research process in the child health setting. However, there are concerns that research involving children ought to be justified and worthwhile, and outweighs any potential harm to the child (Glasper and Ireland, 2000). Casey (2000) examined published primary research studies relating to clinical paediatric nursing between January 1995 and December 1997 in four journals (*Paediatric Nursing, Journal of Advanced Nursing, Child Care Growth and Development, Journal of Child Health Care*). Although she identified that there was a significant increase in the number of published studies over the three-year interval, the majority of studies were small scale, focused upon local need and of doubtful rigour. English and Bond (1998) are clear that children's nurses must avoid becoming obsessed with the academic base of practice, if many of the positive initiatives currently being undertaken are to be further developed (citing the example of the numerous pre-operative preparation schemes for children, which have been developed in the absence of a sound evidence base). Children's nurses may need to focus on the art of nursing, and incorporating best available evidence with best clinical practice, if implementing evidence-based practice is to maintain its current momentum.

Ultimately, it will be the integration of evidence with practitioners' experiences, the context of care delivery and patient wishes that will determine whether nursing practice becomes evidence-based. Cheater and Closs (1997) offer cautionary advice that, at present, it is an unrealistic aspiration for nurses to be able to base all their care on evidence, for no other reason than the lack of available evidence for every nursing activity. In fact, the Nursing and Midwifery Audit Information Service (RCN, 1998) is categorical in its statement that lack of evidence is not a justifiable reason for not providing quality care; clinical decision-making also needs to be based upon reasoning and experience.

References

Audit Commission (1993) *Children First: A Study of Hospital Services.* HMSO, London

Bristol Royal Infirmary (2001) *Bristol Royal Infirmary Inquiry.* Bristol Royal Infirmary, Bristol

Burns LS (1997) Advances in pediatric anesthesia. *Nurs Clin N Am* 32(1): 45–69

Casey A (2000) The role of professional journals in promoting evidence-based care. In: Glasper EA, Ireland L, eds. *Evidence-based*

Child Health Care: Challenges for Practice. Macmillan Press Ltd, London

Chambers N, Jolly C (2002) Essence of care: making a difference. *Nurs Stand* 27(17): 40–44

Cheater FM, Closs SJ (1997) The effectiveness of methods of dissemination and implementation of clinical guidelines for nursing practice: a selective review. *Clin Effect Nurs* 1: 4–15

Clarke J (1999) Evidence-based practice: a retrograde step? The importance of pluralism in evidence generation for the practice of health care. *J Adv Nurs* 8: 89–94

Crombie IK, Davies HTO, Abraham CSC, *et al* (1993) *The Audit Handbook; Improving Health Care Through Clinical Audit*. John Wiley and Sons, Chichester

Department of Health (2003) *Getting the Right Start: National Service Framework for Children. Emerging Findings*. Stationery Office, London

Department of Health (2003a) *Getting the Right Start: National Service Framework for Children. Standards for Hospital Services*. Stationery Office, London

Department of Health (2001) *Learning from Bristol: The Report of the Public Inquiry into Children's Heart Surgery at the Bristol Royal Infirmary 1984–1995*. Stationery Office, London

Department of Health (2001a) *Essence of Care. Patient-focussed Benchmarking for Healthcare Practitioners*. Stationery Office, London

Department of Health (2000) *The NHS Plan. A plan for Investment, A Plan for Reform*. Stationery Office, London

Department of Health (1999) *Government Expenditure Plans 1996–97 and 1998–99*. HMSO, London

Department of Health (1999a) *Hospital Episode Statistics 1997/8*. HMSO, London

Department of Health (1998) *A First Class Service: Quality in the NHS*. HMSO, London

Department of Health (1997) *The New NHS Modern and Dependable*. HMSO, London

Department of Health (1996) *The Patient's Charter: Services for Children and Young People in Hospital*. HMSO, London

Department of Health (1995) *Methods to Promote the Implementation of Research Findings in the NHS: Priorities for Evaluation*. HMSO, London

Department of Health (1994) *The Allitt Inquiry: Independent Inquiry Relating to Deaths and Injuries on the Children's Wards at Grantham and Kesteven Hospital during the period February to April 1991 (Clothier Report).* HMSO, London

Department of Health (1991) *Welfare of Children and Young People in Hospital.* HMSO, London

Department of Health (1976) *Fit for the Future; The Report of the Committee on Child Health Services.* HMSO, London

DiCenso A, Cullum N (1998) Implementing evidence-based nursing: some misconceptions. *Evidence-Based Nurs* 1(2): 38–40

Dixon N (1991) *Medical Audit Primer.* Health Care Quality Quest, Hampshire.

Effective Health Care Bulletin (1999) *Getting Evidence into Practice.* University of York, NHS Centre for Reviews and Dissemination 5 (1)

Effective Health Care Bulletin (1994) *Implementing Clinical Guidelines.* University of York, NHS Centre for Reviews and Dissemination 1(8)

Ellis JM (2000) Sharing the evidence: clinical practice benchmarking to improve continuously the quality of care development. *J Adv Nurs* 32(1): 215–25

Ellis JM (1995) Paediatric benchmarking: a success story. *Value for Money Update* 17: 6–7

Ellis JM, Cooper A, Davies D *et al* (2000) Making a difference to practice: clinical benchmarking part 1. *Nurs Stand* 14 (32): 33–37

Ellis JM, Morris A (1997) Paediatric benchmarking: a review of its development. *Nurs Stand* 12: 43–46

English C, Bond S (1998) Evidence-based practice: easier said than done. *Paediatr Nurs* 10(5): 7–11

Field M, Lohr K (1992) *Guidelines for Clinical Practice: From Development to Use.* National Academy of Sciences, National Academy Press, Washington

Flemming K (1998) Asking answerable questions. *Evidence-Based Nurs* 1(2): 36–37

French P (1999) The development of evidence-based nursing. *J Adv Nurs* 29(1): 72–78

Glasper EA, Ireland L (2000) *Evidence-based Child Health Care: Challenges for Practice.* Macmillan Press Ltd, London

Grimshaw JM, Russell IT (1994) Achieving health gain through clinical guidelines II: Ensuring guidelines change medical practice. *Q Health Care* 4(3): 45–52

Harvey G (1995) Relating quality assessment and audit to the research process in nursing. *Nurse Research Compend* **3**: 203–14

Heath S (1998) *Perioperative Care of the Child.* Mark Allen Publishing, Wiltshire

Hogg C (1994) *Setting Standards for Children Undergoing Surgery.* Action for Sick Children, London

Hopkins A (1995) Some reservations about clinical guidelines. *Arch Dis Childhood* **72**: 70–75

House of Commons Health Select Committee (1997) *Hospital Services for Children and Young People: Fifth Report.* Stationery Office, London

Jones S (2003) Essence of care in a children's hospital. *Paediatr Nurs* **15**(3): 12–13

le May A (2000) *Evidence-based Practice.* Nursing Times Clinical Monographs, 1. Nursing Times Books, London.

McClarey M (1998) Implementing clinical effectiveness. *Nurs Man* **5**(3): 16–19

McSherry R, Haddock J (1999) Evidence-based health care; its place within clinical governance. *Br J Nurs* **8**(2): 113–17

Ministry of Health (1959) *The Welfare of Children in Hospital (Platt Report).* HMSO, London

Ministry of Health (1946) *Report of the Care of Children's Committee (Curtis Report).* HMSO, London

Muir Gray J (2001) *Evidence-based healthcare, how to make health care policy and management decisions,* 2nd edn. Churchill Livingstone, Edinburgh

NHS Executive (1998) *Achieving Effective Practice. A Clinical Effectiveness and Research Information Pack for Nurses, Midwives and Health Visitors.* National Health Service Executive, Leeds

NHS Executive (1996) *Promoting Clinical Effectiveness: A Framework for Action in and through the NHS.* National Health Service Executive, Leeds

Noble RR, Micheli MS, Hensley MA, *et al* (1997) Peri-operative considerations for the pediatric patient: a developmental approach. *Nurs Clin N Am* **32**(1): 1–15

Nursing and Midwifery Audit Information Service (1998) *Levels of Evidence: Information for Clinically Effective Practice.* RCN, London

Paediatric Forum of the Royal College of Surgeons (2000) *Children's Surgery—A First Class Service.* Royal College of Surgeons, London

Royal College of Anaesthetists (1999) *Extremes of Age*. Royal College of Anaesthetists, London

Royal College of Nursing (2000) *Clinical Governance: How Nurses can get Involved*. RCN, London

Royal College of Paediatrics and Child Health (1996) *Children's Surgical Services*. Royal College of Paediatrics and Child Health, London

Sackett D, Straus S, Richardson S, *et al* (1997) *Evidence-based Medicine: How to Practice and Teach EBM*. Churchill Livingstone, London

Sackett D, Rosenberg W, Muir Gray J, *et al* (1996) Evidence-based medicine: what is it and what it isn't. *Br Med J* 312(7023): 71–72

Smith J, Callaghan L (2001) Development of clinical guidelines for the sedation of children. *Br J Nurs* 10(6): 376–83

Thomas LH, McColl E, Cullum N, *et al* (1999) Clinical guidelines in nursing, midwifery and the therapies: a systematic review. *J Adv Nurs* 30(1): 40–50

Thornes R (1991) *Just For the Day*. National Association for Welfare of Children in Hospital, London

Touloukian R (1995) Pediatric surgery between 1860 and 1900. *Journal of Pediatric Surgery* 30(7): 911–16

Woolf S, Grol R, Hutchinson A, Eccles M, Grimshaw J (1999) Potential benefits, limitations, and harm of clinical guidelines. *Br Med J* 318: 527–30

TWO

PRINCIPLES OF CARING FOR THE CHILD AND FAMILY

Children and their families are unique, with complex lives and needs, and are increasingly playing a much more active role in healthcare decision-making processes and participating in treatments. Healthcare professionals need to ensure care is individualised and integrated into everyday practice (Department of Health, 2003; 1996; 1991). This is not easy because there is lack of a shared understanding of the meaning of individualised care, and a poor knowledge or willingness to understand the needs of an increasingly diverse population (Redfern, 1996; Reed, 1992; Waters and Easton, 1999). Gerrish (2000) suggests that individualised care encompasses the principles of respecting individuality and the concept of holism focuses upon need, promotes independence, promotes partnership and negotiation, and ensures equity and fairness. If the health of the child is to be maximised, in addition to addressing specific health problems, broader factors such as the child and family's cultural background, religious beliefs, ethnicity, health beliefs, family structure and functioning need to be considered. This chapter will explore some of these concepts in more detail, with the first section providing an overview of the development of family-centred care and suggesting ways to work more effectively with the child and family. Effective communication with the child and family is paramount within healthcare and will be discussed in section two. Children's rights, consent for treatment and a child's ability to contribute to the decision-making process in relation to his/her healthcare needs, and the ethical and practical issues of restraining children will be the focus of section three. Safeguarding children will be the focus of section four, and section five will consider meeting the child and family's cultural, religious and spiritual needs.

2.1 Parental participation and family-centred care

Early work (Bowlby, 1953; Ministry of Health, 1959; Robert-son, 1958), highlighting the emotional disintegration and plight of children separated from their mothers, culminated in a group of parents, children's nurses and paediatricians advocating that the care of children in hospital should be more humane and family-centred. The slow implementation of the recommendations from the Platt Report (Ministry of Health, 1959) was instrumental in leading a group of parents to establish the National Association for the Welfare of Children in Hospital (NAWCH) in 1961. This actively campaigned for the recognition of the specific needs of the hospitalised child. The re-launch of the society and new name, Action for Sick Children (ASC), in 1991 was timely and coincided with the society reinforcing its beliefs in the ten principles of the Charter for Children in Hospital, originally formulated by NAWCH in 1984 (ASC, 1991). These ten principles are:

- Children shall be admitted to hospital only if the care they require cannot be equally well provided at home or on a day basis

- Children shall have the right to have their parents with them at all times

- Children and/or their parents have the right to information appropriate to their age and understanding

- Children and/or their parents have the right to informed participation in all decisions involving their health care

- Children shall be treated with tact and understanding and their privacy will be respected

- Children shall enjoy the care of appropriately trained staff, fully aware of the physical and emotional needs of each age group

- Children shall be able to wear their own clothes and have their own personal possessions

- Children shall be cared for with children of the same age group

- Children shall be in an environment furnished and equipped to meet their requirements, and which conforms to recognised standards of safety and supervision

- Children shall have full opportunity for play, recreation and education suited to their age and condition.

Involving parents in the care of their sick child should be a core feature of healthcare practice and there is a wealth of literature within nursing journals devoted to this subject. Coyne (1996) and Darbyshire (1993) undertook extensive literature reviews relating to the inclusion of parents in their child's care. The common themes within both papers included:

- The concept of parental participation is ill defined, with a range of terminology used, and little understanding of the terms

- There are extreme variations in the level at which parents participate in care

- Parents often undertake care relating to normal 'mothering tasks', such as bathing and feeding, or non-active roles, such as general supervision of children or comforter roles

- The tasks parents are willing to perform are usually identified in the form of a checklist without any real commitment from nurses to include them in decision-making or negotiation of roles

- There are conflicts between parents and nurses in their perception of parental participation, and between nurses themselves, resulting in confusion and uncertainty for parents

- Much of the care parents undertake is 'assumed' with little negotiation between parents and healthcare professionals

- Parents have many anxieties, including 'parenting in public'

- There are many negative attitudes among nurses towards parents participating in their child's care.

Darbyshire (1993) suggests that, although many nurses welcomed the philosophy of the Platt Report (1959) at the time of its publication, there were others who felt many of its principles challenged the ability of nurses to develop effective relationships with children and provide efficient care. Labelling of parents as 'thick', 'neurotic', 'lazy', or 'troublemakers' was a common occurrence (Darbyshire, 1993) and certainly did not embody the desire to openly welcome parents into the ward environment. Nurses with positive attitudes towards parents and the desire to involve them in the care of their child tended to be senior staff, nurses who had undertaken additional educational programmers relevant to children's nursing and those who were parents themselves. The main conclusions from Coyne (1996) and Darbyshire's (1993) papers include the overwhelming lack of clarity in the concept of parental participation in care, which has been summarised by Darbyshire (1993) as 'one of paediatric nursing's most amorphous and ill-described concepts' (p1672), and the negative view many nurses caring for children have towards parents.

This lack of clarity and common understanding of parental participation in care has resulted in the concept of true partnership as a desirable, but in reality difficult, goal to achieve. There have been attempts to develop a greater understanding and grapple with these concepts. Coyne (1996) undertook a concept analysis in an attempt to describe and understand terminology, such as 'parents in care', 'care by parents' units', 'mutual participation' and 'family-centred care', and how the terminology has changed over time. The earliest description of parents being present with their hospitalised child occurred in the late 1950s in the immediate wake of the Platt Report (1959), where there was a concurrent development of 'rooming-in' facilities. Only the mother's role was considered important and, in general, this was confined to providing emotional support for her sick child.

In the early 1980s, the development of 'care by parents' units' was viewed as the way forward in encouraging parents to assist in the care of their child. However, as Coyne (1996) indicates, the term itself is an anomaly as interpretations were mixed, with many authors stating that parents within these units *could* assist with care (Keane *et al*, 1986; Webb *et al*, 1985) and others advocating a system of active *participation* and parental responsibility (Sainsbury *et al*, 1986). The underpinning philosophy of many 'care by parents' units viewed it as a privilege for mothers to stay and be allowed to undertake tasks delegated by nurses (Webb, 1983), rather than an all-embracing concept involving shared responsibility between the family and nurse for the child's care. However, considering the context in which these changes were taking place, care by parents' units were probably a radical departure from existing models of care provided to hospitalised children and their families. For example, at the beginning of the 1980s, over half the children's wards surveyed had restricted visiting for parents and was a marked contrast with the philosophy of care by parents' units (Thornes, 1983).

Towards the late 1980s, there was a definite desire to move away from the notion that to enable parents to participate in care, a special unit must be developed, and the term 'partnership in care' was beginning to appear in the literature. Fradd (1991; 1987) suggests that, in order to enable families to participate in care, there must be a paradigm shift where parents retain overall responsibility for their child's care and health professionals support parents in the role of caring for their sick child. Again there were subtle changes in the language being used within the literature, such as 'mother' being replaced by 'the family', 'parents' or 'carers'. Most nurses caring for children will be familiar with the 'partnership in care model of paediatric nursing' developed by Casey (1988), which is based upon the underpinning philosophy that the care of children is carried out best by their families, with support from skilled healthcare professional as required. The model operates within the four dimensions associated with nursing: person (or in this case child and family), health, environment and nursing, and the unique relationship between these dimension. Within Casey's model, it is the family's ability to care for the child that is important, with the children's nurses' role complementary to parental care (Casey, 1988). However, there has been a feeling that the progression from parent participation to partnership in care took place in the absence of the essential component of negotiation, and that parents may not have been empowered to take on additional caring roles, but merely expected to do so as delegated by the nurse (Callery and Smith, 1991; Coyne, 1996; Kawik, 1996).

The final term discussed by Coyne (1996) was the model of family-centred care. It is difficult to find a comprehensive definition of family-centred care within the literature. Smith *et al* (2002) suggest that it is 'an all-embracing term used to describe a concept with many different attributes' (p20), but that through common usage it has become a recognised philosophy which underpins the care of the child and family. The critical components of family-centred care are:

- Viewing the family in its social, cultural and religious context whereby in times of stress, family members are not required to conform to norms that are alien to them

- Evaluating individual family members in order to meet their physical and emotional needs and to maximise their ability to care for their child

- Providing explicit information to enable parents to participation in decision-making and the acquisition of knowledge pertaining to their child's illness

- Involving the prime care-giver in developing and evaluating care plans

- Involving families in technical aspects of care, in accordance with their own perceived abilities and willingness to develop the necessary skills

- Continuing usual childcare practices, unless detrimental to the child's well-being, in hospital

- Evaluating the impact of the sick child on the family and taking steps to ensure support continues as needed after discharge, or in the event of death.

(Nethercott, 1993)

Coyne (1996) suggests that the concept of family-centred care has been an evolutionary process that has developed from the concept of mothers rooming in with their hospitalised child.

However, it has been argued that models of care such as 'parental involvement', 'parental participation', 'partnership with parents' and 'family-centred care' co-exist in a hierarchal structure with family-centred care at the pinnacle (Cahill, 1996; Hutchfield, 1999) (*Figure 2.1a*). Smith *et al* (2002) support the position that models of care, relating to parental participation, co-exist and are interrelated; they also suggest that these operate

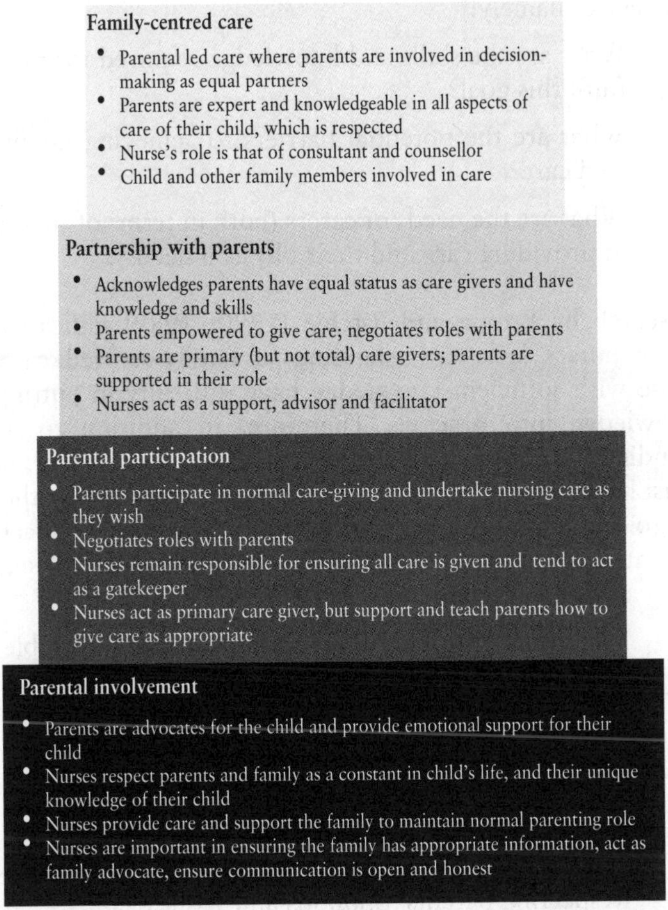

Family-centred care
- Parental led care where parents are involved in decision-making as equal partners
- Parents are expert and knowledgeable in all aspects of care of their child, which is respected
- Nurse's role is that of consultant and counsellor
- Child and other family members involved in care

Partnership with parents
- Acknowledges parents have equal status as care givers and have knowledge and skills
- Parents empowered to give care; negotiates roles with parents
- Parents are primary (but not total) care givers; parents are supported in their role
- Nurses act as a support, advisor and facilitator

Parental participation
- Parents participate in normal care-giving and undertake nursing care as they wish
- Negotiates roles with parents
- Nurses remain responsible for ensuring all care is given and tend to act as a gatekeeper
- Nurses act as primary care giver, but support and teach parents how to give care as appropriate

Parental involvement
- Parents are advocates for the child and provide emotional support for their child
- Nurses respect parents and family as a constant in child's life, and their unique knowledge of their child
- Nurses provide care and support the family to maintain normal parenting role
- Nurses are important in ensuring the family has appropriate information, act as family advocate, ensure communication is open and honest

Figure 2.1a: Hierarchical structure of care in the paediatric setting, indicating main characteristics of each model (adapted from Hutchfield, 1999)

on a practice continuum and, ultimately, it should be the family who choose where they are on the continuum.

Hutchfield (1999) suggests that parental involvement, the lowest denominator in the hierarchy, is the minimal model of care parents can expect. In all probability these boundaries are more fluid than described and individuals may work across these models depending upon their own skills and the experiences and the needs of each family. If children's nurses are aiming to reach the goal of family-centred care, many questions need to be addressed, namely:

- What are the skills and knowledge required for nurses to fulfil this goal?

- What are the potential barriers to achieving family-centred care?

- What are the needs of carers (both in terms of their belief in providing care and their physical needs)?

Research by Brown and Ritchie (1990; 1989) indicated that many nurses lack understanding of family-centred care and those with sufficient knowledge have difficulty in putting this knowledge into practice. Therefore, in addition to understanding the concepts underpinning family-centred care, nurses must have excellent communication skills, in particular the ability to negotiate effectively with families, in order to facilitate parents to participate in their child's care. Neill (1996) suggests this can be achieved by:

- Establishing the level of care parents feel comfortable with and reviewing that level of care over time

- Providing opportunities for parents to express their feelings and concerns

- Taking the lead in providing information

- Assisting parents to make choices

- Respecting parents' opinions and wishes

- Ensuring consistency within the healthcare team, and acting as a mediator between parents and other professionals if necessary

- Involving parents in the nursing process and ensuring parents' physical needs are met.

Bruce and Ritchie (1997) suggest that educational programmes have been addressing knowledge gaps, but there has not been the same emphasis on skills development. Interactive workshops that incorporate families sharing their experiences of caring for a child in hospital could enhance nurses' communication and facilitation skills. Focusing solely upon nurses' knowledge deficits does not address the wide range of phenomena that contribute or hinder the development of family-centred care. There have been some attempts to ascertain parents' views of family-centred care (Callery, 1997; 1997a; Coyne, 1995; Kawik, 1996).

Many of the factors that contribute to promoting effective family-centred care are lacking, especially where family-centred awareness is not evident. The barriers to achieving family-centred care include: poor negotiation between parents and staff; lack of appropriate information; unapproachable staff; and healthcare professionals operating within a paternalistic framework (Neill, 1996). One of the tenets of family-centred care is that the relationship between the family and professionals is based upon mutual respect with non-judgemental, open and honest communication (Hutchfield, 1999). However, there is often an assumption that all families wish to participate fully in the care of their child, implying that a coercive system of involving parents in care may be operating (Coyne, 1995; Smith *et al*, 2002). This can lead to conflicts between healthcare professionals and the family, with eventual breakdown of relationships and disempowerment of the family. During her interviews with parents, Coyne (1995) provided examples where parents were willing to continue complex nursing care, if they already provided this care prior to admission or would learn complex skills necessary to continue care following discharge, but they did not wish to undertake additional nursing skills if these were short-term interventions. Parents expressed high levels of anxiety, which were provoked by undertaking complex tasks and the fear of causing harm to their child. They did not feel that the benefits of learning these complex skills, in the short-term, could be justified.

There are many difficulties placed upon a family when one or both parents are resident, such as financial hardship, organisation of the rest of the family, sleep deprivation and emotional drain. Callery (1997a) explored the cost implications for parents who become involved in their child's care and identified three levels of 'cost': financial, social and personal. Examples of financial costs included:

- Direct loss of income

- Expense of hospital food and drink for themselves and for their child; by being resident, parents often felt pressured into providing substitute food and drinks for their child as standard options were not always appropriate for their child's needs

- Cost of travel

- Cost of making alternative childcare arrangements for other children within the family.

Social costs related to:

- Parents justifying to relatives that the child in hospital was in need of care

- Conflicts between relatives as to who would support siblings; this was often a cause of concern and anxiety for families of a hospitalised child

- Loss of normal social outlets.

Personal costs related to:

- Long periods of boredom

- Periods of intense distress (such as supporting their child through traumatic procedures)

- Extreme feelings of loneliness

- Parents felt isolated

- An inability to maintain normal self-care routines.

Parents did not feel that professionals or other family members had any understanding of the costs of being resident with their child and that it is an emotionally draining experience. Parents found caring adequately for themselves was difficult due to environmental constraints, such as inadequate food (relying on convenience food), lack of facilities or poor facilities for washing and sleeping (Coyne, 1995). Positive support from other resident parents was often a vital lifeline for many.

Despite the barriers, constraints and cost to participating in care, parents appear to be overwhelmingly motivated to stay with their child and do perceive that the psychological benefits to the child outweigh any personal costs (Callery, 1997a; Coyne, 1995; Kawik, 1996). In order for the concepts of family-centred care to be incorporated into practice, there needs to be a commitment to developing the skills and knowledge of nurses and a culture which redresses the balance of power between parents and nurses. Educational programmes need to be geared towards developing skills of nurses caring for children, and nurses themselves need to recognise their own ability in contributing to reducing the barriers experienced by parents. There needs to be wider organisational consideration to address the difficulties families face, such as support mechanisms for parents and accommodation. Policies need to consider cost for parents and there could be much more assistance, such as addressing the type of food available and offering food at staff or non-profit-making rates.

2.2 Communicating with the child and family

Communication has been defined as 'a process that involves a meaningful exchange between at least two people to convey facts, needs, opinions, thoughts, feelings or other information through both verbal and non-verbal means, including face-to-face exchanges and the written word' (Department of Health, 2003a: 1). Mulholland (2003) suggests effective communication is an essential component of quality care and vital in order to:

- Prevent misconceptions and conflicts arising
- Prevent injuries
- Prevent complaints
- Alleviate stress and anxiety.

Effective communication is embedded within the UK Nursing, Midwifery and Health Visitor's Code of Professional Conduct (Nursing and Midwifery Council, 2002).

The national benchmarks within the UK relating to communication between patients, carers and healthcare professionals (Department of Health, 2003a: 2) clearly state that the principles of effective communication are:

- Openness, honesty, common courtesy and transparency
- Consent and confidentiality
- Self-awareness and understanding body language, and other non-verbal communications
- Developing active and empathic listening skills
- Being adaptable and sensitive to language and cultural differences, developmental needs and disabilities, psychological needs and to the context of the communication and situation.

Effective communication is essential if parents are to participate successfully in their child's care (Neill, 1995), and prevent assumptions being made about the nature of their contribution to care (Casey, 1995). In addition to the general principles inherent within ensuring effective communication, Smith *et al* (2002) suggest communication frameworks need to be incorporated into, and become part of, everyday practice. Ahmann (1994) is more critical and suggests nurses caring for children need to (re)learn the communications skill which are necessary to work collaboratively with families. She suggests using either the LEARN framework (Berlin and Fowkes, 1983) or the Nursing Mutual Participation Model of Care (Curley, 1988) because they both shift the focus of communication from the nurse to the child and family. LEARN is an acronym for *listening* to the family's perceptions, *explain* your perceptions as a nurse, *acknowledge* and discuss differences, and *negotiate* agreement about the care delivered. The Nursing Mutual Participation Model's philosophical underpinning relates to the development of communication that facilitates a two-way exchange through open-ended questions.

Effective communication should be embedded in and be a core component of every healthcare intervention (Department of Health, 2003a). Healthcare professionals caring for children will need to refine their communication skills according to the child's age and stage of development, and the context of the interaction (Deering and Cody, 2002; May, 1999). The general principles of effectively communicating with children include:

- Positioning at the same level as the child and making eye contact
- Finding out about the child's interests, but avoiding making the child feel self-conscious
- Not 'talking down' to children
- Maintaining a calm, gentle, unhurried manner
- Linking information-giving to daily activities will give a sense of meaning to younger children
- Effective listening
- Not excluding children from conversations
- Discouraging parents from speaking on behalf of their child
- Using language that is appropriate for the child's age
- Using play; it is an important form of communication for children.

In addition, healthcare professionals must apply their knowledge of child development to their communication strategies (Deering and Cody, 2002). For example:

- Infants first communicate through touch, sight and hearing. Cuddling infants and speaking in soft soothing sounds will make them feel more secure

- Although young children have developed rapid language acquisition, they need time to complete their thought processes. Communication should be unhurried to prevent the child becoming frustrated and feeling undervalued. Constructive choices and directing the young child to alternative behaviours are more effective than criticising a young child for any inappropriate behaviours

- School-age children are rapidly developing the ability to use logic and analyse situations, and will form their own (mis)perceptions of a situation. It is therefore important to identify any preconceptions and provide information that is simple, straightforward and factual. In addition, the school-age child may not want to communicate his/her own needs and feeling, and may respond to suggestions of how other children would normally behave in a given situation

- Adolescents have intense feelings and may react to events and people in extreme terms. They may find it difficult to develop trusting relationships with adults. It is important to take time to build a rapport with an adolescent. Listening to their views and having a non-judgemental and straightforward approach are vital. Issues such as consent and confidentiality, and limits (such as a duty to share information that threatens their well-being) need to be discussed.

Play is the medium through which young children express themselves and is a characteristic of healthy, normal childhood. Vital information can be gained about children's perceptions of their environment, their understanding of situations and their feelings through engaging them in and watching them play (May, 1999). The rights for children to have access to suitable play, recreational and educational activities have been embodied within policy documents relating to the care of children in hospital (Department of Health, 2003b; Department of Health,

1996; Department of Health, 1991). The use of play can be a valuable tool, allowing children to become familiar with and explore equipment in a safe and secure environment. Despite the lack of, and inherent difficulties with, research involving children and play, children do value play within the hospital setting and have identified it as a means of reflecting up issues and expressing feelings (Carroll, 2002). The importance of play cannot be overestimated (Webster, 2000) and the benefits within the hospital environment include:

- Introduces normality into a strange environment

- Lessens the impact of anxiety

- Facilitates the expression of fears and experiences

- Provides a safe outlet for using up energy

- Helps reduce boredom and waiting times

- It is satisfying for the child to achieve something

- Provides opportunities for meeting other children, which offers companionship and support

- Facilitates the preparation of treatments and procedures

- Can be used as a medium for children to perform tasks relating to their treatment.

In order to enhance the therapeutic effect of play, activities should be constructed in an appropriate manner and consider the child's age and capabilities, while recognising any limitations as a result of the hospitalisation (Webster, 2000). Healthcare professionals working with children will need to be familiar with the types of play, particularly those suitable for therapeutic uses (medical play, projective play, role play, distraction techniques) and the way in which play changes as the child develops (solitary, parallel, onlooking, being sociable, simple operative and complex co-operative play) (*table 2.2a*). Play specialists are vital members of the healthcare team caring for children and can lead specific therapeutic play interventions, while contributing to and directing the development of hospital play services. In the perioperative setting, there is opportunity to develop structured play activities in relation to preparation for hospital admission, procedures, the theatre experience and advanced preparation of post-operative care.

Table 2.2a: Social development of play (adapted from Wong and Perry 1998)

Age	Developmental stage	Play activities
0–2 years	**Solitary Play** Plays on own, and self-absorbed	Young infants enjoy and are rewarded by interactions with people Activities should stimulate the senses; bright, noisy, tactile toys and using different mediums, such as water and sand, are suitable
2–3 years	**Parallel Play** Plays alongside others, but does not share. Will defend own play things	Physical skills are developing, therefore push-pull toys, shape fitting and repetitive activities are suitable
3 years	**Onlooking Play** Shows greater interest in others, but does not attempt to join in	Activities can be conducted as a group. However, each child will work on his/her own activity
3–5 years	**Sociable Play** Tries to join in and be accepted; social talk may not be related to the play activity	Make-believe and unrestricted physical activities are suitable May enjoy basic tasks (errands and helping adults
5 years onwards	**Simple Co-operative Play** Shares, takes turns and divides play activities into tasks	Imaginative play, dressing up are suitable Continuation of school activities, such as reading and writing skills
8 years onwards	**Complex Co-operative Play** Concerned with the content of play; complex and definite roles and rules	Clubs, games, hobbies, being with peers are important

2.3 Children's rights and consent to treatment

Children's rights

When considering the rights of children, a distinction needs to be made between legalities and moral rights. A legal right is an entitlement, which is acknowledged and enforced by an existing law. There are legal rights that apply to children. A moral right is a claim to a right, and in the case of children is usually bestowed upon them by adults. Legal and moral rights relating to children are implicitly linked to the general beliefs a society has about children. Franklin (1995) suggests that members of a society are divided into two broad categories, namely childhood and adulthood, with the passage into adulthood synonymous with rights, privileges and obligations. Archard (1993) states the concept of childhood varies between and within societies in terms of the years childhood lasts, the qualities that distinguish the child from the adult and, subsequently, the significance of these differences. In Britain, adulthood corresponds with the age of majority (18 years). A child's experiences upon reaching 18 years of age will be unique and inherently diverse, consequently the range of skills, competencies and abilities to enable them to confront various situations will be extremely individualised. However, it is usually adults within a society that determine when children are deemed able to participate in decision-making processes. Franklin (1993) describes three philosophical perspectives that influence society's views relating to a child's rights: paternalism, interventionism and libertarianism.

Paternalism results in choices being made for children on their behalf, usually by their parents. This is based upon the premise that children are irrational, lack adult reasoning and knowledge, and do not posses the cognitive capacity to make reasoned and informed decisions. Children are perceived as vulnerable and therefore require adults to secure their welfare. This assumes adults are capable of making rational, autonomous decisions not only for themselves, but also on behalf of their children (Archard, 1993). Interventionists believe that there are certain times when professionals should assume the responsibility of decision-maker, in order to decide a child's best interests. This has the same basic premise as paternalism; however, the power balance has shifted to healthcare professionals. In fact children view healthcare professionals as interventionists and in general feel they are unsupportive and not really interested in exploring their needs (O'Quigley, 2000).

Libertarians believe that children are capable of making informed choices and that, like adults, children will make mistakes based upon their decisions. Inevitably, it would be through participating that children would learn through experiences. There are certainly flaws with a libertarian approach in that a very young child will have an obvious incapacity to exercise his/her rights (Archard, 1993). The debate relating to whether a child has the ability to make his/her own decisions is circular;

namely, what age is childhood and is age a valid criterion for the attribution of rights. Libertarians would argue that it is a mistake to judge a child's ability to participate in the decision-making processes solely on age. Other considerations are of vital importance, such as level of competence and previous experiences.

The move towards a libertarian view has been reflected in the 1989 United Nations Convention on the Rights of the Child (Freeman, 1995; Newell, 1993). Article 12 of the Convention is a clear statement of a libertarian philosophy and is particularly pertinent to a child's right to consent to treatment:

> *'the child who is capable of forming his or her own views has the right to express those views freely in all matters affecting the child: the views of the child being given due weight in accordance with age and maturity of the child'* and *'the child shall in particular be provided with the opportunity to be heard in any surgical or administrative proceedings affecting the child directly; or through a representative body.'*

The principle of involving children in the decision-making process had been previously adopted within the United Kingdom. It certainly appears to be a key component within the *Children Act* (Department of Health, 1989) and *Working Together to Safeguard Children* (Department of Health, 2000). Subsequent guidance relating to children, such as *The Patients' Charter: Services for Children and Young People in Hospital* (Department of Health, 1996), *Children's Surgery—A First Class Service* (Paediatric Forum of Royal College of Surgeons, 2000) and *The Reference Guide to Consent for Examination or Treatment* (Department of Health, 2001) indicate the need to involve children in decisions made about their healthcare. If children are to participate in the decision-making process relating to their healthcare needs, strategies must be developed to help children access information at a level appropriate to their level of understanding. This will require a concerted effort to listen and understand a child's point of view. Successfully listening to children requires:

- Providing adequate information in order for the child to express his/her views

- Allowing children to tell the whole story without interrupting

- Using a non-intrusive style of communication; remaining open-minded and non-judgemental

- Viewing children's abilities and competencies as being different from rather than lesser than those of adults

- Being alert to signs of distress in the child

- Respecting that some children will not want to be involved in decision-making

- Having an awareness of developmental and cultural factors affecting each individual child

- Assuring confidentiality (or clearly identifying limits).

(O'Quigley, 2000)

Consent

Consent is required from a patient, of any age, before medical treatment can be given (Department of Health, 2001). Treatment that involves touching without consent can constitute assault. Consent can be expressed or implied. Expressed consent is when the patient has clearly and explicitly expressed that treatment can proceed, either verbally or in writing. It is usual practice for healthcare professionals to obtain written consent for invasive procedures. Implied consent is indicated by the patients' behaviour. Issues surrounding a child's ability to consent for treatment and contribute to the decision-making process in relation to his/her healthcare needs are complex and multifaceted. Dilemmas for healthcare professionals in relation to obtaining consent for surgery in children include:

- The young child who is unable to understand the implications of the treatment

- The child who has sufficient ability to understand the nature and implications of medical treatment and is therefore in a position to consent for treatment

- The child who has sufficient ability to understand the nature and implications of medical treatment, but refuses to consent for treatment

- The parent who declines to give consent despite the treatment being deemed necessary for the health of the child.

These situations will be considered in the context of the current law in England, Wales and Northern Ireland. Major differences in the law for Scotland will be highlighted. In relation to consent in children, healthcare professionals must understand who may have parental responsibility. Parental responsibility refers to:

- Legal parents, in other words the child's biological parents. However, both parents do not necessarily have parental responsibility; parental responsibility applies to both the mother and father if they were married at conception, birth or some time after birth. If the parents have never married, the mother alone has parental responsibility, although a father can apply for parental responsibility

- The child's legally appointed guardian

- A local authority authorised person, who has been designated parental responsibility in a care order in respect of the child

- A local authority authorised person, who has holds an emergency protection order in respect of the child.

(Department of Health, 1989)

In England, Wales and Northern Ireland there is no statute that gives children under 16 years of age the right to consent to treatment (British Medical Association, 2001). According to the Family Law and Reform Act, 1969, (sub section 8 and 22(2)), the person with parental responsibility must provide consent for any medical treatment on behalf of a minor (a child under 16 years of a age). Statute in Scotland is slightly different in that the

Age of Legal Capacity (Scotland) Act, (1991) applies, which states:

> '*a person under the age of 16 years shall have legal capacity to consent on his own behalf to any surgical, medical or dental treatment where, in the opinion of a qualified medical practitioner attending him, he is capable of understanding the nature and possible consequences of the procedure or treatment*'

(section 2(4))

Children can legally consent to surgical, medical or dental treatment at or over 16 years of age; in England, Wales and Northern Ireland, the Family Law and Reform Act, 1969, sub section 8 and 22(2) applies and in Scotland the Age of Legal Capacity Act, 1991, section 1(1)b and 3(3)e applies. These laws were reaffirmed in the section concerning children and young people, within the Department of Health's recently published reference guide relating to consent for examination or treatment (Department of Health, 2001). This is a statutory right and has the same standing as consent given by an adult. It is not necessary to obtain consent from a parent or guardian. There are exceptions to this statutory right, which include minors of 16 years or older, who are deemed incapable of consenting for treatment due to 'disability'. Unfortunately, there is no attempt to define disability or how to assess capability. Consent for treatment is not necessary in life-threatening situations. Children can consent to treatment at any age provided that they are deemed to have sufficient understanding and intelligence to fully understand treatments being proposed (Gillick v West Norfolk and Wisbech Area Health Authority, 1985, All ER 402). In many ways the Gillick case, in which a mother failed in a challenge to prevent her daughter from being able to have the contraceptive pill prescribed without her knowledge, was a landmark case for advocates of child rights and became case law. Those with parental responsibility cannot override this decision, although the decision can be overridden by a court of law.

On the surface, it appeared that the Gillick case would resolve many of the uncertainties relating to children's ability to consent to treatment. Unfortunately, two major issues emerged; how do you assess a child's competence and does the Gillick principle apply to refusal of treatment? In some ways, case law has addressed issues relating to a child's right to refuse medical treatment, which does not follow Gillick principles. It is obvious that the law views ability to consent for treatment and ability to refuse treatment as two distinct issues. If a child refuses medical treatment, the decision can be overridden by the person with parental responsibility for that child and by the court, even if the child has sufficient understanding of his/her actions and the subsequent consequences of these actions (Re W, 1992; Re E, 1993). It must be noted that the one test case that has occurred in Scotland concerning a child's refusal to treatment resulted in the Sheriff concluding that logically, if a child was declared competent, this should apply to both consent and refusal to treatment and was adequately covered in the 1991 Age of Legal Capacity (Scotland) Act (British Medical Association, 2001).

Competence is a difficult issue and a crucial component when considering the ability of a child to consent to treatment. Spencer (2000) suggests it is issues surrounding competency that results in ethical dilemmas for health professionals working with children, partly because of difficulties in defining and assessing competence. Orr (1999: 292) defines competence as 'an ability to understand and decide about a choice of actions'. Understanding competence requires making assumptions about a child's cognitive level. Probably the most widely applied theories relating to the cognitive development of children are those of Piaget (Santrock, 1998), which are based upon the premise that children acquire cognitive competence according to a universal sequence (Appendix I). According to Piaget's Stages of Cognitive Development, children who have reached the end of the formal operational stage (about 15 years of age) are capable of hypothetical deductive reasoning. In other words, adolescents have the cognitive ability to develop hypothesis about ways to solve problems and can systematically deduce the best course of action, while younger children do not have these abilities. From a cognitive perspective, it could be assumed that an adolescent is competent to consent or refuse healthcare and the younger child is not. However, it is vital to consider socio-cultural factors and the individual uniqueness of development in order not to underestimate a child's ability to reason and deduce (Archard, 1993; Donaldson, 1978; Santrock, 1998).

Healthcare professionals have a duty to protect children from actual or potential harm (Department of Health, 1989; Nursing and Midwifery Council, 2002). This may result in dilemmas for those caring for children, if a parent declines to give consent despite the treatment being deemed necessary for the health or even survival of the child. An example would include children of parents who are Jehovah's Witnesses, who may not consent to treatment if this necessitates giving blood products. In the case of Jehovah's Witnesses, consent for treatment for a child requiring non- urgent surgery where there is a likelihood of blood products being required can be obtained from a court of law by making the child a ward of court (Ashley, 1997). Catlin (1997) suggests that this should not be viewed as an extreme course of action and may be in the best interests of the family. If parents are coerced to sign a consent, which includes giving blood products in opposition to their religious beliefs, there is the potential for that family to be ostracised from their church, wider family and friends. This is not acting in the best interests of the child and family. However, removing that decision-making process from the family may be a satisfactory solution, in that parents cannot be held responsible.

In addition, with modern technology and advances in anaesthesia the need to administer blood products can be avoided. Ashley (1997) has summarised best care as:

- Clearly identifying which blood products the family will accept

- Establishing potential risks and communicate these to the family

- Advanced planning of procedures to ensure the child is in optimal health state for surgery, including consideration of timing of operation, surgical techniques and type of procedure

- Surgery and anaesthesia conducted by experienced surgeons

- Considering the use of pre-operative erythropoietin for major surgery
- Considering the need to undertake major surgery in stages to reduce potential blood loss.

Ashley (1997) suggests that the thoughtful planning of surgery, in order to minimise blood loss for patients who are Jehovah's Witnesses, should be universally applied. This may be particularly pertinent in the current climate, where there is increasing concern relating to the risk of bloodborne infections following the administration of blood products. Autologous blood transfusions are not usually acceptable to Jehovah's Witnesses because the blood has lost contact with the body. In the case of a child requiring a blood transfusion in an emergency situation, the British legal system would uphold the decision to administer blood products without parental consent (Ashley, 1997). Examples where parents have been deemed not to act in the best interests of the child include the well-documented case of a baby with Down's syndrome who required surgery. The child's parents believed the natural course for their child was a short life span and did not wish treatment to proceed (Re: B, 1981). The courts did not support the parents' wishes, deeming that the best interest for the child was to undergo surgery.

The dilemmas relating to consent in childhood arise from attitudes society have towards children, individuals' professional values and beliefs, and lack of clarity within the legal framework. If these issues are to be resolved, children's views need to be understood and respected, which can only be achieved if they are consulted. There is a paucity of research that directly relates to a child's ability to consent to treatment and even less that has directly involved children in the research process. Alderson (1993) undertook a comprehensive study that examined a child's *ability to arrive at informed, wise decision about surgery* (p3). Her findings indicated:

- Young children (eight years and above) are able and wish to share in discussions with healthcare professionals about their treatment

- Distress was reduced when the children's views were considered
- Children felt that preparation for experiences that would occur following surgery was vitally important
- Participation increased the confidence of the young person and facilitated better trust with healthcare professionals.

Healthcare professionals interviewed believed it was difficult to put a definite age on competence and that occasionally children as young as five or six years of age could have some understanding and make complex decisions. The majority of children within the study did not want to be the sole decider of their care, but they did wish to share decision-making with their parents and, in general, the children were cautious about how much decision- making they wish and could cope with. It is perhaps difficult to accept that there is a difference between having the right to choose and choosing the right action when it comes to the care of children.

Restraining children

Many procedures, such as venepuncture and cannulation, dressing changes and radiography, necessitate the child remaining motionless, which requires healthcare professionals and the child to work co-operatively. If the child refuses to co-operate and the procedure is deemed in his/her best interests, the application of restraint is the usual end point. Until recently, healthcare professions have accepted the practice of restraint as a necessary component of caring for children (Jeffery, 2002; Lambrenos and McArthur, 2003). Awareness of the rights of the child (Newell, 1993) and legislation that clearly places the child's welfare at the centre of care (Department of Health, 1989) and the proliferation of guidance from professional bodies (British Institute of Learning Disabilities, 2001; Department for Education and Employment, 1998; Department of Health, 2001a; Department of Health, 1993; Royal College of Nursing, 2003) has resulted in the restraining of the child becoming an uncomfortable practice (Lambrenos and McArthur, 2003).

The Department of Health (1993) considers physical restraint to be the positive application of force with the explicit intention of overpowering the child. Implicitly this occurs without the child's consent. The Royal College of Nursing guidelines relating to restraining, holding still and containing children and young people (Royal College of Nursing, 2003) adopt this definition, but differentiate between restraint and holding still, where holding still is a method of assisting the child to remain motionless with his/her consent for a given procedure. It is therefore distinguished from restraint by the force required and the intention.

Bland *et al* (2003) have described the potential ability of benchmarking as a way of implementing and monitoring good practice in relation to procedural restraints. The principles of good practice in relation to restraining and holding still include:

- Ensuring the necessity of the procedure

- Ensuring restraint is the last option

- Preparing the child adequately for any procedure

- Respecting the rights of the child

- Involving parents and carers in the decision-making process and the actual procedure

- Identification of alternative methods to restraint and offering choices in relation to methods used, such as using splints and swaddles

- Considering ethical and legal issues

- Openness and an ability for all staff to express concerns

- Policies appropriate to client group and care setting

- Staff training in restraining techniques and alternatives, such as distraction

- Physical restraints are never used in a way that could be considered indecent

- Allowing opportunity for debriefing.

    (Bland *et al*, 2003; Royal College of Nursing, 2003)

2.4 Safeguarding children

The Department of Health (2003c) and the Royal College of Nursing (2003a) clearly identify that everyone who works with or comes into contact with children has a duty to safeguard and promote their well-being. The *Children Act* (Department of Health, 1989) was designed to promote the interests of children, setting out the principles that ensure their welfare and protection, with the two documents *Working Together to Safeguard Children* (Department of Health, 2000) and *Framework for the Assessment of Children in Need and Their Families* (Department of Health, 2000a) providing detailed strategies for implementing policy into practice. *Working Together to Safeguard Children* (Department of Health, 2000) outlines the wider issues in relation to safeguarding children, and includes:

- Working with and supporting the family in meeting the needs of the child, including keeping them safe and free from harm

- Proving additional support for the child with special needs and assisting the family to enable the child to reach his/her full potential

- Ensuring a wide range of services, in particular educational, social and health, is available so that each child has maximal opportunities to develop. Ensuring effective co-ordination, communication and collaboration between agencies and professionals with responsibility for children

- Having rigorous processes in place to be followed when there are concerns about a child being at risk or having suffered significant harm.

Unfortunately, the essence of the *Children Act* (1989) has become primarily associated with child protection issues. This is understandable in the context of the number of high-profile child abuse inquiries over the last 30 years (the most well-known children within the UK include Maria Colwell 1973, Jasmine Beckford 1985, Tyra Henry 1987, Kimberley Carlile 1987, Victoria Climbie 2000). Despite the increasing expectations that healthcare professionals inform their clinical decisions on the best available evidence (Thompson *et al*, 2001), the repetitive content, particularly ineffective communication between professionals and an inability to address recommendations, within these reports is disappointing. Laming (2003) poignantly described widespread organisational malaise, when reporting on the (lack of) actions of professionals concerned with protecting Victoria Climbie.

The Royal College of Nursing's (2003a) guidance paper *Child Protection—Every Nurse's Responsibility* suggests nurses are well placed to identify and safeguard the child at risk from harm, which requires nurses to be able to recognise the child at risk and be clear about their own roles and responsibilities in relation to putting the child's needs first. Although there is no definitive sign, symptom or injury that constitutes abuse, general indications of child abuse may include:

- Physical signs (slap marks, unusual bruising, bite marks)
- Poor physical care, inadequate hygiene, inappropriate dress, failure to seek medical advice
- Unrealistic parental expectations/overprotection
- Changes in behaviour/withdrawal/fear/heightened anxiety/self harm
- Inconsistencies in reporting injuries
- Repeated attendance with a variety of injuries and in different healthcare settings.

(Royal College of Nursing, 2003a: 4)

In all situations, it is the context of each sign, symptom or injury that is important. It is vital that any concerns relating to a child's welfare are raised, documented and followed up. The Department of Health's (2003c) guidance document for children's services, *What To Do if You Are Worried a Child is Being Abused,* outlines the principal stages of child protection procedures, from raising concerns through to the child protection conference and ongoing follow-up, which are represented in a series of easy-to-follow flow-charts. The principles within the guidance clearly identify the need for effective communication and sharing information in the context of safeguarding and promoting the welfare of children. Although being familiar with the guidance and local organisation policies and procedures is essential, nurses must understand their roles and responsibilities within the process (Royal College of Nursing, 2003a). This requires an understanding of the issues and potential conflicts relating to confidentiality, professional and ethical codes when working with the child and family.

Nurses are bound by their Code of Professional Conduct (Nursing and Midwifery Council, 2002); this ensures that the public are protected through professionally agreed standards related to the care they receive. Furthermore, nurses are personally accountable for their acts and omissions 'regardless of advice or directions from another professional' (Clause 1.3; Nursing and Midwifery Council, 2002). This both implicitly and explicitly identifies that the professional nurse's responsibilities lie with the child. The increased roles of specialist nurses, and of statutory and voluntary organisations, with the central aim of better collaboration and ensuring that the child remains paramount, as outlined in the *Children Act* (Department of Health, 1989) have led to professional colluding, a criticism of child protection case conferences and investigations (Department of Health, 1995; Laming, 2003). Although it is important to explore and understand differing viewpoints, collusion is always destructive (Lawrence, 2002), whether it is between professionals or between the professional and the 'family', and this may be where the best intentions become flawed. If the child's needs are paramount in decision-making, it should not occur.

Dependent upon your moral thinking, do you take the Kantian approach and do the right thing (Beauchamp and Childress, 2001) or do you offer the greatest happiness to the maximum number of people (Mill, 1986)? These dilemmas are constant within child protection and thus clinical decisions are never easy. There are inherent difficulties in incorporating pure ethical principles within child protection, as the complexities within each case negate this approach. However, philosophically, the governing moral principle should be that the child's needs are paramount. The complex issues relating to ethical dilemmas could be best served by the use of supportive clinical supervision, where ethical issues could be debated in relation to practice. The Beckford Report (London Borough of Brent, 1985) and the Carlile Report (London Borough of Greenwich, 1987) linked the failure in the performance of both health visitors and social workers in relation to child protection, with inadequacies in the professional supervision provided by the field worker's superiors. It was deemed that clinical supervision should be proactive rather than reactive, resulting in guidance for senior nurses, health visitors and midwives (Department of Health and Social Security, 1988). The guidance clearly stated that 'autonomy' should not lead to 'isolation'.

Issues relating to clinical autonomy can be linked to the area of confidentiality, which is often one of the biggest stumbling blocks for many practitioners. Practitioners are increasingly concerned about losing the trust of their clients/patients if they disclose information gained in 'confidence'. There is no conclusive evidence to support this 'feeling'. As a general rule, information gained should be treated as confidential. However, and most importantly, there will be no breach of confidentiality if consent has been gained to share information, whether it be written or verbally given. Part of every nurse's best practice should include highlighting to patients/clients that there may be times when there is a need to share information with other professionals, both within the healthcare team and other agencies, in order to provide appropriate care delivery (Department of Health, 2002; Department of Health, 2000). A supportive, trusting professional relationship will be fostered if the boundaries are clearly and openly set from the outset (Clause 2.3; Nursing and Midwifery Council, 2002). Policies, including those relating to obtaining consent, should be aimed at protecting the individual, while supporting the practitioner. Furthermore, policies should not hinder the process of protecting children. Clause 5 of the Code of Conduct (Nursing and Midwifery Council, 2002) clearly states the impracticalities of continually seeking consent every time there is a need to share information. However, if consent is refused, and in order to ensure the child's needs remain central to any decision-making process, disclosure may be necessary and appropriate (Department of Health, 1989; Nursing and Midwifery Council, 2002).

Additional concerns may arise when considering case law legalities (precedence built up over a period of time) relating to the Common Law Duty of Confidence, where information shared between a client and a professional (such as the patient/doctor relationship) is expected to be kept in confidence. Nevertheless, this duty is not absolute and disclosure can be justified when there is overriding public interest, such as cases of actual/suspected child abuse (Department of Health, 2003c). This is validated by the Code of Conduct (Nursing and Midwifery Council, 2002) clause 5.3, where there is a duty to protect the patient/client from the risk of significant harm. Further clarification is contained within the Data Protection Act (Great Britain; Parliament 1998a), where it is very clear that data protection is overridden when:

- There are particular concerns for the welfare of the child
- The information is to be disclosed to social services or another professional
- The disclosure can be justified under the Common Law Duty of Confidence.

The Human Rights Act (Great Britain, Parliament 1998), which incorporates the European Convention on Human Rights, article 8, recognises the right for privacy in family life, but is once again not absolute. Disclosing confidential information to protect a child may cause considerable disruption to a person's private life. However, Article 8(2) can justify this if it is necessary to prevent crime or to protect the health and welfare of the child.

In order for nurses to play their part effectively in protecting the child, they need to consider how they interpret and use policies to support their everyday practice. The relationship between the nurse and the family needs to be established upon professional roles and responsibilities, albeit in an empathetic and compassionate manner, rather than 'befriending families' within a more social type of relationship. A relationship based on friendship may result in influences within the relationship that have the potential to cloud future judgments (Lawrence, 2002). This is a balance requiring the nurturing and development of specific skills relating to working with families, particularly developing effective, clear, frank and appropriate communication skills.

2.5 Providing holistic care; meeting the cultural, religious, and spiritual needs of children

Culture, religious and spiritual beliefs are probably among the most powerful forces that shape human experiences (Rehm, 2000) and can provide comfort, strength and help support families during periods of stress and illness. Attending to all dimensions of care, including cultural, religious and spiritual needs, is vital to the overall well-being of the child (Anderson and Steen, 1995; Kenny, 1999). Therefore healthcare professionals must have an understanding of the broad principles of these concepts.

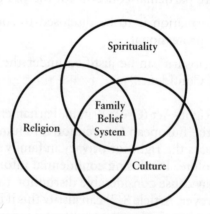

Figure 2.5a: Inter-relationship between culture, religion and spirituality

For many families, health belief systems (*Figure 2.5a*) will be influenced by cultural, spiritual and religious beliefs. Although interrelated, for ease each area will be considered separately.

Culture and healthcare needs

There are diverse interpretations of the term culture. Leininger's (1995) definition of culture as 'the learned and shared beliefs, values and lifeways of a designated or particular group which are generally transmitted intergenerationally and influence one's thinking and action modes' is probably the most universally accepted (p9). There are limitations with this definition, including:

● Lack of recognition of the political and economic factors that influence culture

● Lack of recognition of the complex interplay with spirituality and religion

● Implications that culture is static

● Failure to recognise inter-generational changes can lead to the stereotyping of individuals.

(Whiting, 1999)

The advantage of Leininger's (1995) definition is the deliberate exclusion of terms, such as race, ethnicity and religion. Although these terms may be inextricably linked, the definition acknowledges that not all cultures are based upon racial and ethnic identity. Examples of subcultures include physical ability, occupation, educational attainment, socio-economic status, and sexual preference or identity.

Cultural issues have a considerable impact upon health. Within the UK, low socio-economic status or belonging to a minority ethnic group (Acheson, 1998; Alexander, 1999), or both (Gerrish, 1999), has considerable impact upon health and well-being. Minority ethnic groups are likely to have higher unemployment and are much more likely to be reliant on income support, both of which contribute to higher levels of poverty within these groups compared with the majority of the population. The NHS Plan (Department of Health, 2000b) reiterated that the healthcare system in the UK will continue to be based upon the principles of providing access to all. The plan identified the need for welfare authorities to work together to debate issues that contribute to poor health and ensure that the health needs of all cultures are being addressed. Within the UK, one in four children belongs to a non-white, minority ethnic group (Department of Health, 2003c). The distribution of ethnic groups is not evenly reflected throughout the country, with many large urban areas having over 40 percent of their population from a minority ethnic background. There is considerable evidence highlighting the failure of the National Health Service to provide care that meets the health needs of minority ethnic groups (Acheson, 1998; Alexander, 1999).

In order to provide and deliver healthcare effectively to diverse cultures, there needs to be an understanding of their specific healthcare needs and their beliefs relating to health issues, and removal of the potential barriers within organisations that prevent services being culturally sensitive. Minority ethnic groups will have different health needs from the dominant culture and, in general, will only have access to services based upon Western ideologies. Certain diseases' conditions are more frequent within cultural groups; sickle cell disease in African populations, cystic fibrosis in Caucasian populations, Tay-Sacks disease in Jewish populations, neural tube defects in British populations and thalassemia in Mediterranean populations. Although there may be similarities in healthcare problems, and therefore many existing services are appropriate (Acheson, 1998), the organisation of these services can be a barrier to providing effective care to ethnic groups. Gerrish (1999: 1269) suggests that minority groups suffer a 'double jeopardy' in that not only does the inverse care law apply, where those who need care most receive the least in terms of resources, but in addition the services provided do not meet their needs. Vydelingum studied the experiences of South Asian patients within an acute healthcare setting and found that many organisational constraints, such as inadequate translation services, lack of appropriate food, lack of facilities for private prayer, inflexible visiting hours, poor communication about care given, lack of discharge planning, feelings of isolation and loneliness, significantly affect the quality of the healthcare experience for minority ethnic groups (Vydelingum, 2000). These negative experiences will undoubtedly influence future decisions relating to accessing services.

Healthcare practitioners need to explore ways in which they can contribute to improving services for minority ethnic groups (Gerrish, 1999; Vydelingum, 2000). If not, health disadvantages and discrimination experienced by minority ethnic communities will continue to occur.

The perceived cause of illness and impact upon the child and family may vary greatly between cultures (Whiting, 1999). For example, the notion of promoting independence is a Western ideology and for some cultures (for example, South Asian communities) dependence may not be viewed negatively, where there are expectations that more able members of a family will provide the care needed. It may be more appropriate to provide healthcare to support the family in their role to provide care, rather than in gaining independence for the individual. However, within all cultures, it is vital not to make stereotypical judgements (Gerrish, 1999) and, although there is a need to exhibit cultural flexibility as part of the care delivered, it is of vital importance to value each client as an individual (Rasool, 1995).

Although lacking in clarity, the term 'culturally competent care' is gaining popularity within healthcare literature (Kim-Godwin et al, 2001). They suggest three components are necessary if culturally competent care is to become a reality: cultural knowledge, cultural sensitivity and cultural skills. Cultural knowledge is the cognitive understanding of other cultures (Kim-Godwin et al, 2001). It is impractical and inappropriate for healthcare professionals to have detailed knowledge about every culture. It may be more appropriate for healthcare professionals to focus upon gaining an in-depth knowledge of one or two of the cultures, which form the majority of the client group they care for (Leininger, 2001). This knowledge should be used to establish trust and prevent destructive practices.

Cultural sensitivity is the affective aspect of care and is concerned with respecting other cultures (Kim-Godwin et al, 2001). This includes respecting gender role differences between cultures, family roles and child-rearing practices, use of appropriate touch, cleanliness and hygiene practices, dietary differences, and rituals relating to death and dying (Josipovic, 2000). It also involves being flexible and focusing upon the client's needs, maintaining an open attitude and willingness to listen to the child and family and to learn from them (Leininger, 2001). A starting point could be to develop a deep understanding of your own culture's values, beliefs and practices, which should help prevent cultural clashes and racism (Leininger, 2001; Zoucha, 2000).

Cultural skills are the practical skills required to ensure cultural needs are being met (Kim-Godwin *et al*, 2001). This begins by determining health needs through skilled assessment of the cultural identities and particular beliefs of the child and family, and incorporating these into care delivery (Rehm, 2000). There are an increasing number of specific cultural assessment tools, but these are time-consuming and difficult to apply in practice (Whiting, 1999). Therefore healthcare professionals may feel more comfortable adapting existing models, which usually contain a cultural component. Models such as 'the partnership in care model' developed by Casey (1988) could be applied more effectively to ensure the child and family's cultural needs are identified (Whiting, 1999).

The importance of effective communication skills has been highlighted as one of the most important factors in providing quality care (Josipovic, 2000). Achieving effective communication when there are language barriers imposes additional challenges. Josipovic suggests that there is a lack of interpreters for many cultural groups. Other options, such as encouraging nurses to develop fluency in a second language that reflects the local population (resourced appropriately) and introduction of languages in nursing programmes (although with current demands upon curricula this may be difficult), are potential ways forward (Josipovic, 2000). Non-verbal communications and styles of communication are vital and can assist in gaining the trust of a child and family; for example, certain gestures and body positioning acceptable in one culture may be offensive within other cultures.

Religious beliefs

Anderson and Steen (1995) advocate that the assessment of the child and family should include details of their religious beliefs and how these beliefs are practised to ensure that planned care can include all aspects of a child's normal routines. Johnson (1998: 5) defines religion as 'any system of beliefs regarding the cause, nature and purpose of the Universe, especially belief in or worship of God or gods'. However, many people identify themselves as belonging to a religious group not necessarily because they have strong religious convictions, but more as a way of identifying their particular lifestyle and specific practices in relation to activities of living (such as food and hygiene choices) and rituals of death and dying (Neuberger, 1994). This is important for healthcare professionals because the recording of denominational affiliation alone does not provide any information about the relevance of religion or the religious practices for the individual child and family. Religious beliefs are often central to perceptions of health and illness (Johnson, 1998). For example, attitudes towards the role of healthcare professionals, the role of alternative medicines, euthanasia, organ donation, disposal of the body and burial rituals will be influenced by religious beliefs. Neuberger (1994) suggests it is important for healthcare professionals to have some understanding of the religious traditions of their patients in order to provide appropriate and sensitive care. The underpinning philosophies of those religions more commonly encountered are summarised, as an encouragement to further, more specific reading.

The three main Western religions are Christianity, Islam and Judaism (Carson, 1989). Sikhism is the fourth most followed, monotheistic religion, and is important due to the increasing number of Sikhs living in the United Kingdom. Although monotheism is the major belief in Western philosophy, there are many different practices within these religions.

Christianity

Christianity, the most followed Western religion, was founded upon the principles that Jesus, who is proclaimed to be the Son of God, embodied God (the creator of heaven and earth) in a human form. He was crucified for the sins of humanity, resurrected and ascended to heaven. Christians believe in following the example of Jesus, a loving and just person, and in an afterlife that can be a place of perfect existence (Heaven) or a place of torment (Hell). Of the festivals, Christmas (celebrating the birth of Jesus) and Easter (celebrating the Resurrection) are the best known. Unfortunately, this may be more to do with their secularisation and financial exploitation.

The diversity within Christianity (for example Roman Catholicism, Orthodox Christianity, Presbyterianism, Protestant Church and Seventh Day Adventism) and different cultures which practise the Christian faith make generalisations in relation to Christian customs, such as baptism, confession, Holy Communion and last rites, difficult (Christmas, 2002; Papadopoulos, 2002). It is not only important to consider the division of Christianity practised, but the importance of religious beliefs for each individual. Belief in an afterlife influences the views Christians may have towards illness and death. This can vary from a positive approach, where if there is a feeling that the path of Jesus has been followed then life after death will hold no fears, to a negative one, where others may view illness and death as a punishment from God and may experience feelings of anger and disillusionment. In the case of a sick child, it may be vitally important for the parents to have the child christened.

Islam

After Christianity, Islam is the second most followed religion, and is the religion of the Muslim people. Originating about 1400 years ago, it has swiftly become a world faith. Islam is much more than a religious faith; it is a system of belief that influences social and legal systems, and governs family life, law and order, ethical codes, dress and cleanliness codes. The Islamic faith believes in one true God—Allah—and, although there have been earlier messengers—Adam, Noah, Abraham, Moses and Jesus—Allah chose Mohammed, the final messenger, to reveal the Islamic faith to the world, and its intent of achieving peace and security. All Muslims accept the teachings of the Koran (the holy writings) and observe the five duties of Islam: faith, prayer performed ritualistically five times a day, fasting, giving alms to the poor, and pilgrimage to Mecca. Ramadan is an important period for Muslims and represents the month in which Allah revealed the Holy Koran to the prophet Mohammed. The two most important celebrations are

Eid-ul-Fitr (which marks the end of Ramadan) and Eid-ul-Adha (which celebrates Mohammed's pilgrimage from Mecca to Medina in order to escape persecution). Friday is a holy day for Muslims.

Muslims have a strong desire for modesty (nakedness is extremely offensive) and may find assistance with personal activities during illness humiliating. Muslims wash with running water before prayers and after using the toilet. Hospital settings are not always accommodating in provisions for cleansing practices (Akhtar, 2002). In general, Muslims will eat all types of fruits, grains and vegetables, certain types of fish (with scales), poultry and some meat products. Muslims will not eat pork and pig products and shellfish. The most important consideration for Muslims is the way in which food and particularly meats are prepared. This not only refers to the process of slaughtering animals, but the whole process of food production, which should follow Islamic laws and customs; food prepared in this way is known as 'Halal'. Consumption of alcohol is deemed offensive. After death, Muslim family members usually stay with the body, pray and perform all rites and ceremonies. Muslims prefer non-Muslims not to touch the body (Akhtar, 2002). Where possible burial should occur within 24 hours.

Judaism

Judaism has a complicated history and is largely a religion of a people, the Jews, who regard Abraham as the founder of Judaism. Abraham made a historic journey to Canaan (now modern Israel), where he settled with his people. Generations later, during the great famine, his descendants travelled to Egypt to look for food where they were 'enslaved'. Moses led them from slavery in search of the Promised Land. The implications of these journeys are very significant to Judaism. All Jews have a strong attachment to Israel, the holy city of Jerusalem and the sacred texts. Judaism has many sub-divisions, often based upon racial origins, each having differences in beliefs and practices. Orthodox Jews follow the original teachings and traditions of the faith closely according to the sacred texts. At the opposite end of the continuum of Judaism are the non-Orthodox Jews, who have adapted their faith and customs by incorporating

69

modern theories about Judaism into everyday life. All Jews believe that humans are made in the image of God and should try to seek holiness in every part and activity of life, that obeying the 'law' is doing God's will, and in the Messiah. The Messiah will be a person specially anointed by God and will come to the world in order to bring an era of peace.

The main festivals within Judaism include: Rosh Hashanah (New Year), Yom Kippur (the holiest day in which every individual is judged by God) and Passover (an eight-day festival commemorating the freeing from slavery with ritual foods eaten). During prayer, Jewish males traditionally wear a skullcap and small boxes containing sacred passages tied on with leather straps. Male Jewish children are circumcised on the eighth day after their birth. Naming the child occurs at this ceremony. At the age of 13, Jewish law considers boys to have reached adulthood, marked by the Bar Mitzvah service held in honour of being permitted to read from the sacred texts for the first time. The comparable ceremony for girls is a Bat Mitzvah. Jewish dietary laws include not eating certain foods, such as pork and certain seafood, or meat unless the blood has been removed (kosher), and not mixing dairy and meat products at the same meal. These laws also include how animals must be slaughtered so as to minimise suffering. Traditionally, Jews do not perform any work on the Sabbath (sundown on Friday until sundown on Saturday), which is spent in prayer and religious study. In relation to healthcare treatment, medical advice would be followed. Termination of medical treatment and organ donation will be difficult areas because of the value placed upon life (Collins, 2002). Upon death, the body should be prepared in a specific manner, ritually washed and placed in a coffin for burial, generally the day after death. Where possible, the family's rabbi should be involved in death rituals.

Sikhism

Sikhism is the youngest of the world's most followed monotheistic religions. Guru Nanak founded Sikhism in the fifteenth century. Born a Hindu, he and his followers were disillusioned and offended by the contemporary features of Hinduism, particularly the caste system and the power of the priesthood. The aim was a return to religious beliefs that valued the relationship between each individual and God, the search for a virtuous life and that doing 'good' is the only true salvation. The view that Sikhism is a branch of Hinduism is very offensive to Sikhs. The five symbols of the Sikh faith are: uncut hair worn in a bun by both men and women, a comb used to hold the hair up, a steel bangle which is never removed, a dagger worn at all times, traditional knee-length underpants or shorts. Removing these items can be very distressing for Sikhs. Sikhs have a tradition of private prayer and reading the scriptures. There are many Sikh festivals or holy days; the most important is the celebration of Guru Nana's birthday and usually lasts three days.

Many of the lifestyles of Sikhs follow Hindu practices. Where possible, Sikhs shower in a morning prior to private prayer. In general, the only food restriction is not eating meat unless it is halal, with vegetarianism being popular. Alcohol consumption and tobacco smoking are not tolerated. Death may be viewed positively, as Sikhs believe in reincarnation and that the good done in this world affects how the next life will be. As a mark of respect, family and friends will want to visit a sick relative (Gill, 2002). The family will wish to perform last rites and prefer the body to be cremated within 24 hours.

Eastern religious beliefs are influenced by the four main philosophies of Buddhism, Hinduism, Confucianism and Taoism (Carson, 1989).

Hinduism

Hinduism is the name given to a family of ancient religions and cultures that began and still flourish in India. All Hindus believe that the individual soul exists in a cycle of birth, followed by death and then rebirth. Therefore, the principles of Hinduism relate to this cycle; whether one is reborn into a better life, a worse life, or even to live as an animal depends upon the value of one's 'soul' (known as Karma), which is determined by good or bad deeds performed in the current life. The eventual stage of this cycle and therefore ultimate aim for Hindus is to become free from rebirth altogether by attaining liberation. Hindus do not separate religion from other aspects of their existence; Hinduism is a complete approach to life that involves social class, earning a living, family, politics and diet. Hindus believe that living a moral and religious life contributes to an overall well-being and prevents illness. Lifestyles that maximise health, such as regular diet, sleep, defecation, cleanliness and moderate exercise, are advocated. Hindus may wish to discuss these issues with healthcare workers, but will appreciate privacy and care delivered by a healthcare professional of the same sex. Historically, the caste system has been an important feature of the Hindu way of life and traditionally there has been little tolerance for people from a different caste. This may have implications for the positioning of children in a ward environment. Hindus believe in a Divinity or supreme God that is present in everything and, unlike many faiths, do not insist on there being one 'truth' or one 'God' but embrace a wide range of beliefs. There are many Hindu festivals with their origins in the acts of the Gods. The importance of each festival will depend upon the principal God each individual worships.

Hindus believe in purification of the body and mind; practices include: daily washing with running water, washing hands and rinsing the mouth prior to and after meals, private prayer and meditation. Strict cleanliness when preparing food is essential and the more traditional Hindu will only eat food prepared by Hindus of the same caste. An increasing number of Hindus are vegetarian. Beef, which includes avoiding any other food or utensils that have prepared food having had any contact with beef, is forbidden. Periods of fasting are practised. Hindu beliefs and practices vary widely and this includes customs relating to death and laying out of the body. However, most Hindus accept death as part of the life cycle. Relatives will grieve openly with the use of gestures, touch and open mourning. It is important, where possible, for relatives to spend time with the dying person and offer respect (Jootun, 2002) to that relative. There would be strong objections to a post-mortem.

Buddhism

Buddhism as a religion originated about 2500 years ago and has a worldwide following. Siddhartha Gotama, who later became known as Buddha, was the founder of Buddhism. He was born a royal prince in northern India who in his late 20s realised that wealth and luxury did not guarantee happiness. After exploring different teachings, religions and philosophies, he finally found the path to happiness, which included: leading a moral life, being mindful and aware of thoughts and actions, and developing wisdom and understanding. Buddhism is more a philosophy or 'way of life' than a religion, and is an attempt to understand the purpose to life, injustice and inequality around the world, and provide a code of practice or way of life that leads to true happiness. Buddhists believe in 'Karma', the principle that every cause has an effect and the importance of all individuals being responsible for their past and present actions. The eventual stage of this cycle, and therefore its ultimate aim, is to reach a state of infinite perfection. Buddhism acknowledges many gods but it is Buddha himself and his guiding principles that are held in reverence. Buddhist believe in the four noble truths; that life and suffering are intrinsically linked, that suffering is caused by desire, eliminating desire reduces suffering and the way to end suffering is through having the right aspirations, actions and purpose to life. The following principles form the eight doctrines within which Buddhists try to live their life:

- To acquire a complete understanding of life
- To develop the right outlook on life and motives for living
- To practise the 'right' speech, for example no lying, slandering and gossip
- To carry out perfect conduct, being and doing good, not being dishonest and deceitful, never taking a life
- To earn a living in an appropriate manner
- To be self-disciplined
- To develop awareness of self and others through meditation, and to encourage warmth, love and peace
- To develop complete enlightenment through meditation.

There are many special or holy days held throughout the year by the Buddhist community, but Buddha Day is the most important. Practices common to all Buddhists include: meditation, vegetarianism, and acceptance of the human life cycle. From a healthcare perspective, devout Buddhists may not wish to be administered opiates or sedatives as these may cloud the senses (Northcott, 2002). Accepting death and preparing for death will often be in a calm manner. Organ donation will be viewed positively because it is an opportunity to help others (Northcott, 2002). There are no elaborate rituals after death. The body should be wrapped in a sheet without any emblems and be cremated.

Perhaps some of the most complex belief systems occur amongst the Chinese people. This is partly because of the co-existence and fusion of the major philosophies of Buddhism, Confucianism and Taoism, the turbulent history of China, and the separation of religion by social class, which all have impacted and influenced the Chinese way of life. Confucianism is more than a religion; it is a social and ethical system and dates back to the sixth century bc. Its philosophical underpinnings are based upon establishing social values, institutions and the ideals of the traditional Chinese society, in order to establish a social order. These philosophies are balanced with developing an understanding of humanity and living a harmonious life by valuing everyday life, treating each other with love and respect, and considering the needs of all. Although Confucian teachings have now been abandoned, it has been a dominant way of life in China for centuries and its philosophies impact upon the Chinese way of life.

Taoism

Laoze founded the Taoism philosophy, believing that society, power and wealth were a fallacy, and that the basis of a stable society would be through the development of an inner sense and living harmoniously with nature. Taoist ideals and images inspire a love of nature and an intensity for life, including health and well-being, vitality, longevity and even immortality. Therefore, there has been a natural tendency to associate Taoism with herbal medicine and natural therapies, macrobiotic cooking, massage and exercise. Many Taoists believe that there are a myriad of spirit gods (good and bad), which encompass both the natural world and the internal world of the human body.

A characteristic of the Chinese peoples' religious beliefs has been the ability to incorporate new beliefs with old traditions and rituals. Therefore many festivals, such as Chinese New Year, are closely tied with 'folk religion' and are celebrated whether Buddhist or Taoist. As many Chinese people fuse the three major religious philosophies that have traditionally existed in China, understandably, religious and lifestyle practices are diverse and very individualised. All Chinese people will have a strong belief in the family, as this is where the moral and ethical codes of a society begin. There is also the general belief in a continuation of life after death. Death may be viewed as a natural event and preparing for death will be important to the individual and family. Rituals relating to impending death and handling the body vary considerably depending upon individual beliefs.

The extent to which individuals practise their religious faiths is highly variable. It is vital that healthcare professionals find out the child and family's preferences in order to provide care sensitive to individual needs. Lifestyle restrictions and rituals can be ascertained from undertaking a detailed assessment during admission to hospital. In addition, and with the family's permission, it may be beneficial in times of stress to contact the hospital chaplaincy services or relevant spiritual leaders, for guidance and to offer support to the child and family.

Spirituality

Casey's (1988) partnership model embodied the need to take a holistic approach to the care of children, recognising that there will already exist a health belief system within the family. The model identifies the child as a unique functioning, growing and developing individual, and in order to achieve their potential in areas of physical, emotional, cognitive and spiritual development, they require protection, support and nurturing. Reference to the spiritual needs of children is a key feature within policy documents, philosophies and standards relating to the care of children (Action for Sick Children, 1991; Department of Health, 2003; Department of Health, 1991; Department of

Health, 1989; Royal Collage of Nursing, 1994). However, these are often represented as banal statements with limited guidance in relation to incorporating the spiritual needs into practice. Although there is a growing body of literature relating to the spiritual needs of the child, the meaning of spirituality in childhood, in common with the concept in general, is poorly understood.

There is no real consensus or indeed authoritative definition as to what constitutes spirituality (Narayanasamy, 2001). It would seem that spirituality is an umbrella term or 'catch all' phrase for anything that is not material or physical in origin (Cobb, 2001). The debates surrounding spirituality have led to the concept being subjective, confusing and polarised. At one end of the continuum, spirituality is viewed synonymously with religion, while at the other spirituality applies to all people, irrespective of a faith or belief in a god/deity and is a universal phenomenon applying to all, believers and unbelievers alike (Burnard, 1988; Cawley, 1997). Spirituality has been described in terms of:

- Existentialism, the need to find meaning and purpose in life (Frankl, 1987)

- A source of connectedness or interconnectedness within oneself, with other people, and the Universe at large (Reed, 1992a)

- A universal phenomenon located within all people, primarily coming into focus during time of crisis (Murray and Zentner, 1989)

- Different meanings to different people depending upon their worldview or own philosophy of life (Martsolf and Mickley, 1998).

Within child health, understanding the concepts relating to spiritually needs to consider the child's cognitive development, which will affect how a child expresses spiritual needs (Ratcliff, 1995). Smith and McSherry (2003) undertook a concept analysis with the aim of providing examples of how children express spiritual beliefs and identifying the implications for clinical practice (*Figure 2.5b*).

Figure 2.5b: Examples of how children express spiritual beliefs, linked to Erikson's (1963) stages of child development (adapted from Smith and McSherry, 2003)

Erikson's stages of psychosocial development	Key features	Examples of children's expressing spiritual beliefs
Stage I Trust vs mistrust (first year of life	A sense of trust develops through an infant feeling physical comfort and having basic needs met, such as feeding. This stage of development and interaction forms the prototype for the future relationships and life expectations. A tentative link is made between the support parents provide to an infant by developing trust, with the ability to foster spiritual well-being.	Due to limited ability to influence their environment or communicate on a linguistic level, it is difficult to identify an infant's spiritual needs. However, Bradford (1995) suggests that hopes and fears are aspects of spirituality, and positive experiences can be fostered in a child through love and affection, security and a stimulating environment.
Stage II Autonomy vs shame and doubt (late infancy and toddlerhood)	After gaining trust in the care givers, infants discover that their behaviour is their own and begin to assert their sense of independence or autonomy; they realise their will. If restrained too hard, they develop a sense of shame and doubt.	A three year old was describing what happens when a person dies:'people who die go to prison'. 'This little boy was an avid watcher of the "A-team", where lots of "bad guys" were blown up as a matter of routine, and somehow end up in prison' (Pfund, 2000: 145). In this case, there is a link between illness and death, with punishment and wrongdoing. Pfund highlighted the importance of understanding this little boy's perceptions of death (his brother was terminally ill) and the need to facilitate understanding that illness is not due to a wrongdoing.
Stage III Initiative vs guilt (pre-school years)	The child experiences a challenging, widening social world where active, purposeful behaviour is needed to cope with these challenges. Children begin to assume responsibility for their bodies, their behaviour, their toys and their pets. Developing a sense of responsibility increases initiative. Guilt and anxiety may arise if the child is reprimanded too harshly for irresponsible behaviours.	Steen and Anderson (1995: 10) highlight a four year old's hospitalisation: 'Jason slept very little the night of his hospital admission. The nurse brought in his breakfast tray and set it on the bed-side table in front of him. Before anyone realised what was happening Jason pushed the tray of food off his table and on to the floor.' There may be a link here between Jason's spiritual distress, fears and anxiety, which are being exhibited through disruptive behaviour.

Erikson's stages of psychosocial development	Key features	Examples of children's expressing spiritual beliefs
Stage IV Industry vs. inferiority (junior school years)	Children's initiative brings them into contact with a wealth of new experiences; they direct their energy towards mastering knowledge and intellectual skills. If suppressed, there is a danger of the child feeling inferior, unproductive and incompetent. This natural need for knowledge can be fostered and developed.	Mary, a nine year old, demonstrated mastery of knowledge; however, she also reflects upon this knowledge and applies it to herself when considering a neighbour's misfortune: 'I saw a neighbour, and he'd been in an accident, and he told my dad that he'd just as soon die later because of all the pain he has. The funny thing—our neighbour, he smiles, despite his troubles. He's glad he can see the sun come up in the morning, my mom says. Today I saw the sun coming up, and I was glad, and I thought, I should be double glad, because I can see it, and I love the way the whole sky becomes light up, presto, and I don't have any pain' (Coles, 1990: 134). In many ways this is a powerful representation of self-awareness.
Stage V Identity vs identity confusion (adolescence)	Individuals attempt to find out who they are and where they are going. Adolescents are faced with many new roles, romantic, vocational, which they need to explore in a healthy manner and should be neither pushed nor restricted, otherwise identity confusion may occur.	Haroon, 11 years old, was being bullied at school and had prayed to Allah to give him strength: 'when I was at school, I looked the bully in the eye, and was ready to take him on. Maybe he would have won if we'd fought, but I was ready to test him, and with that he lost interest in me. It was Allah who had given me strength' (Coles, 1990: 70).

It is doubtful that healthcare professionals consider the spiritual needs of children, its meaning to children, its changing appreciation as the child develops and the impact of not considering this aspect of a child's needs. Ebmeier *et al* (1991) suggest that there is a relationship between stress and activation of spiritual needs. This is particularly pertinent in children, where it is accepted that the hospital experience is stressful for the child, and that children bring with them a range of preconceived ideas, existing fears and fantasies, and concerns about separation from familiar surroundings, social isolation and death. Pfund (2000) suggests that children experience many traumatic life-threatening events (illness, death, abuse) and like adults will draw upon all previous experiences, including religious and spiritual beliefs, in an attempt to make sense and cope with crisis. However, in general, children will have much more limited experiences and their developmental stage may have a direct impact upon the interpretation of their experiences. Seden (1998) suggests that practitioners can respond to a child's spiritual needs by:

- Ensuring a child-centred approach to care that enables children to express their beliefs

- Developing an understanding of the multifaceted nature of spirituality

- Understanding that spirituality may be expressed in religious beliefs

- Taking advice from religious communities as appropriate

- Being aware and utilising available training packages.

Within nursing, Anderson and Steen (1995) suggest the basis for all care (including spiritual) is the nursing process, which must inevitably have assessment as the starting point. Omitting spiritual assessment may deny a child the opportunity to maintain normal home routines (an important component of child healthcare) and does not foster a respect for the family beliefs. Spiritual stress will not be recognised and there will be difficulties in planning individual care in response to a child's distress. Anderson and Steen (1995) suggest that assessment of spiritual concerns should include both the child's and family's concepts of faith, sources of strengths and hopes, and the relationship between beliefs and health. The assessment can only be achieved if practitioners have an understanding of the complexities of spirituality and are willing to listen and interpret the child's and family's views.

References

Acheson D (1998) *Department of Health Report: Independent Inquiry into the Inequalities in Health.* Stationery Office, London

Action for Sick Children (1991) Working together for change. *Cascade: 1* ASC, London

Age of Legal Capacity (Scotland) Act (1991) section 2(4), section 1(1)b and 3(3)e

Ahmann E (1994) Family-centred care: shifting orientation. *Pediatr Nurs* **20**(2): 173–76

Akhtar S (2002) Nursing with dignity, Part 8: Islam. *Nurs Times* **98**(16): 40–42

Alderson P (1993) *Children's Consent to Surgery*. Open University Press, Buckingham

Alexander Z (1999) *Department of Health Report: Study of Black, Asian, and Ethnic Minority Issues. Independent Inquiry into the Inequalities in Health*. Stationery Office, London

Anderson B, Steen S (1995) Spiritual care reflecting God's love to children. *J Christian Nurs* **12**(2): 12–17, 47

Archard D (1993) *Children Rights and Childhood*. Routledge, London

Ashley E (1997) Anaesthesia for Jehovah's Witnesses. *Br J Hosp Med* **58**(8): 375–80

Berlin EA, Fowkes WC (1983) A teaching framework for cross-cultural health care. *West J Med* **139**(6): 934–38

Beauchamp TL, Childress FM (2001) *Principles of Biomedical Ethics*. Oxford University Press, New York

Bland M, Bridge C, Dixon D *et al* (2003) Procedural restraint in children's nursing: using clinical benchmarks. *Prof Nurse* **17**(12): 712–15

Bowlby J (1953) *Child Care and the Growth of Love*. Penguin, Harmondsworth

Bradford J (1995) *Caring for the Whole Child: A Holistic Approach to Spirituality*. The Children's Society, London

British Institute of Learning Disabilities (2001) *Code of Practice*. BILD Publications, Kidderminster

British Medical Association (2001) *Consent, Rights and Choices in Health Care for Children and People*. BMJ Publishing Group, London

Brown J, Ritchie J (1990) Nurses' perceptions of parents and the nurse's roles in caring for hospitalized children. *Children's Health Care* **19**: 28–36

Brown J, Ritchie J (1989) Nurses' perceptions of their relationships with parents. *Mat-child Nurs J* **18**: 79–96

Bruce B, Ritchie J (1997) Nurses' practices and perceptions of family-centred care. *J Pediatr Nurs* **12**(4): 214–22

Burnard P (1988) The spiritual needs of atheists and agnostics. *Prof Nurse* Dec 130–32

Cahill I (1996) Patient participation. *J Adv Nurs* **24**: 561–71

Callery P (1997) Caring for parents of hospitalized children: a hidden area of nursing work. *J Adv Nurs* **26**: 992–98

Callery P (1997a) Paying to participate: financial, social and personal costs to parents of involvement in their children's care in hospital. *J Adv Nurs* **25**: 746–52

Callery P, Smith L (1991) A study of role negotiation between nurses and parents of hospitalized children. *J Adv Nurs* **16**: 772–81

Carroll J (2002) Play therapy: the child's views. *Child Family Soc Work* **7**: 177–87

Carson VB (1989) *Spiritual Dimensions of Nursing Practice*. WB Saunders Philadelphia

Casey A (1995) Parnership nursing: influences on involvement of informed carers. *J Adv Nurs* **22**: 1058–62

Casey A (1988) A partnership with child and family. *Sen Nurse* **8**(4): 8–9

Catlin A (1997) Commentary on Johnny's story: transfusing a Jehovah's Witness. *Pediatr Nurs* **23**(3): 316–17

Cawley N (1997) Towards defining spirituality. An exploration of the concept of spirituality. *Int J Pall Nurs* **3**(1): 31–36

Christmas M (2002) Nursing with dignity, Part 2: Christianity I. *Nurs Times* **98**(11): 37–39

Cobb M (2001) *The Dying Soul: Spiritual Care at the End of Life*. Open University Press, Buckingham

Coles R (1990) *The Spiritual Life of Children*. Harper Collins, London

Collins A (2002) Nursing with dignity, Part 1: Judaism. *Nurs Times* **98**(9): 33–35

Coyne I (1996) Parent participation: a concept analysis. *J Adv Nurs* **23**(5): 733–40

Coyne I (1995) Partnership in care: parents' views of participation in their hospitalized child's care. *J Clin Nurs* **4**: 71–79

Curley MA (1988) Effects of the nursing mutual participation model of care on parental stress in the pediatric intensive care unit. *Heart Lung* **17**(6): 682–98

Darbyshire P (1993) Parents, nurses and paediatric nursing: a critical review. *J Adv Nurs* **18**: 1670–80

Deering CG, Cody DJ (2002) Communicating with children and adolescents. *Am J Nurs* **102**(3): 34–41

Department for Education and Employment (1998) *Guidance on Section 550A of The Education Act: The Use of Reasonable Force and Control or Restraint of Pupils.* HMSO, London

Department of Health (2003) *Getting the Right Start: National Service Framework for Children. Emerging Findings.* Stationery Office, London

Department of Health (2003a) *Essence of Care. Patient-focused Benchmarks for Clinical Governance.* Stationery Office, London

Department of Health (2003b) *Getting the Right Start: National Service Framework for Children. Standard for Hospital Services.* Stationery Office, London

Department of Health (2003c) *What To Do If You Are Worried a Child is Being Abused.* Stationery Office, London

Department of Health (2002) *Delivering the NHS Plan.* Stationery Office, London

Department of Health (2001) *The Reference Guide to Consent for Examination or Treatment.* Stationery Office, London

Department of Health (2001a) *Valuing People: A New Strategy for Learning Disabilities for the 21st century.* Stationery Office, London

Department of Health (2000) *Working Together to Safeguard Children.* Stationery Office, London

Department of Health (2000a) *Framework for the Assessment of Children in Need and Their Families.* Stationery Office, London

Department of Health (2000b) *The NHS Plan: A Plan for Investment, A Plan for Reform.* Stationery Office, London

Department of Health (1996) *The Patient's Charter: Services for Children and Young People in Hospital.* HMSO, London

Department of Health (1995) *Messages from Research.* HMSO, London

Department of Health (1993) *Guidance on Permissible Forms of Control in Children's Residential Care.* HMSO, London

Department of Health (1991) *Welfare of Children and young People in Hospital.* HMSO, London

Department of Health (1989) *The Children Act.* HMSO, London

Department of Health and Social Security (1988) *Guidance for Senior Nurses Health Visitors and Midwives.* DHSS, London

Donaldson M (1978) *Children's Minds.* Fontana, USA

Ebmeier EC, Lough MA, Huth MM, Autio L (1991) Hospitalized school children express ideas, feeling and behaviors towards God. *J Pediatr Nurs* 6(5): 337–49

Erikson EH (1963) *Childhood and Society*. 2nd edn. WW Norton, New York

Family Law and Reform Act (1969), sub section 8 and 22(2)

Fradd E (1991) An invitation to influence change. *Paediatr Nurs* 3(7): 6–8

Fradd E (1987) A child alone. *Nurs Times* 83(42): 16–17

Frankl V E (1987) *Man's Search for Meaning: An Introduction to Logotherapy*. Hodder and Stoughton, London

Franklin B (1995) *The Handbook of Children' Rights; Comparative Policy and Practice*. Routledge, London

Franklin B (1993) *The Rights of Children*. Blackwell, Oxford

Freeman M (1995) Children's rights in a land of rites. In: Franklin B, ed. *The Handbook of Children's Rights; Comparative Policy and Practice*. Routledge, London

Gerrish K (2000) Individualised care: its conceptualization and practice within a multiethnic society. *J Adv Nurs* 32(1): 91–99

Gerrish K (1999) Inequalities in health care provision: an examination of institutional influences on the provision of district nursing care to minority ethnic communities. *J Adv Nurs* 30(6): 1263–71

Gill BK (2002) Nursing with dignity, Part 6: Sikhism. *Nurs Times* 98(14): 39–41

Gillick v West Norfolk and Wisbech Area Health Authority (1985) *All England Report 402*

Great Britain Parliament House of Commons(1998) *Human Rights Act 1998* c.42. Stationery Office, London

Great Britain Parliament House of Commons (1998a) *Data Protection Act 1998* c.29 Stationery Office, London

Hutchfield K (1999) Family-centred care: a concept analysis. *J Adv Nurs* 29(5): 1178–87

Jeffery K (2002) Therapeutic restraint of children: it must always be justified. *Paediatr Nurs* 14(9): 30–33

Johnson E (1998) Integrating healthcare and spirituality: considerations for ethical and cultural sensitivity. *Maryland Nurse* 17(5): 5

Jootun D (2002) Nursing with dignity, Part 7: Hinduism. *Nurs Times* 98(15): 38–40

Josipovic P (2000) Recommendations for culturally sensitive nursing care. *Int J Nurs Pract* 6(3): 146–52

Kawik L (1996) Nurses' and parents' perceptions of partnership and participation for a hospitalized child. *Br J Nurs* 5(7): 430–34

Keane S, Garralda ME, Keen JH (1986) Resident parents during paediatric admissions. *Int J Nurs* 23(3): 247–53

Kenny G (1999) The iron cage and the spider's web: children's spirituality and the hospital environment. *Paediatr Nurs* 11(5): 20–23

Kim-Godwin YS, Clarke PN, Barton L (2001) A model for the delivery of culturally competent community care. *J Adv Nurs* 35(6): 918–25

Lambrenos K, McArthur E (2003) Introducing a clinical holding policy. *Paediatr Nurs* 14(4): 30–33

Laming PB (2003) *Victoria Climbie Inquiry*. Stationery Office, London

Lawrence R (2002) Collusion: A concept analysis. *Comm Practition* 75(4): 135–38

Leininger M (2001) A mini journey into transcultural nursing with its founder. *Nebraska Nurse* 32(2): 16–17

Leininger M (1995) *Transcultural Nursing: Concepts, Theories, Research and Practices*. 2nd edn. McGraw Hill, New York

London Borough of Brent (1985) *A Child in Trust: The Report of the Panel of Inquiry into the Circumstances Surrounding the Death of Jasmine Beckford*. London Borough of Brent, London

London Borough of Greenwich (1987) *A Child in mind: Protection of Children in a Responsible Society. The Report of the Commission of Inquiry into the Circumstances Surrounding the death of Kimberley Carlile*. London Borough of Greenwich, London

Martsolf DS, Mickley JR (1998) The concept of spirituality in nursing theories; differing world-views and extent of focus. *J Adv Nur* 27: 294–303

May L (1999) I've got a tummy ache in my head. *Paediatr Nurs* 11(2): 21–23

Mill JS (1986) *On Liberty*. Prometheus Books, New York

Ministry of Health (1959) *The Welfare of Children in Hospital* (*Platt Report*). HMSO, London

Mulholland H (2003) Is your message getting through? *Nurs Times* 99(16): 16–17

Murray RB, Zentner JB (1989) *Nursing Concepts for Health Promotion*. Prentice Hall, London

Narayanasamy A (2001) *Spiritual Care: A Practical Guide for Nurses and Health Care Practitioners*. 2nd edition. Quay Books, England

Neill SJ (1996) Parental participation 2: findings and implications for practice. *Br J Nurs* 5(2): 110–17

Nethercott S (1993) A concept for all the family, family centred care: a concept analysis. *Prof Nurse* 8(12): 794–97

Neuberger J (1994) Caring for Dying People of Different Faiths. 2nd edn. Mosby, King's Lynn

Newell P (1993) *The United Nations Convention and Children's Rights in the UK.* National Children's Bureau, London

Northcott N (2002) Nursing with dignity, Part 2: Buddhism. *Nurs Times* 98(10): 36–38.

Nursing and Midwifery Council (2002) *Code of Professional Conduct.* NMC, London

O'Quigley A (2000) *Listening to Children's Views.* Joseph Rowntree Foundation, York

Orr FE (1999) The role of the paediatric nurse in promoting paediatric right to consent. *J Clin Nursi* 8: 291–98

Paediatric Forum of the Royal College of Surgeons (2000) *Children's Surgery—A First Class Service.* Royal College of Surgeons, London

Papadopoulos I (2002) Nursing with dignity, Part 2: Christianity II. *Nurs Times* 98(12): 36–37

Pfund R (2000) Nurturing a child's spirituality. *J Child Health Nurs* 4(4): 143–48

Rasool GH (1995) The health status and health care of ethno-cultural minorities in the United Kingdom: an agenda for action. *J Adv Nurs* 21(2): 1025–29

Ratcliff D (1985) The development of children's religious concepts: research review. *J Psychol Christian* 4(1): 35–43

Redfern S (1996) Individualised nursing care: its meaning and practice in a general setting. *Nurs Times Res* 1: 22–23

Re: B (a minor) Wardship; medical treatment (1981) 1 Weekly Law Report 1421.

Re: E (a minor) Wardship; medical treatment (1993) Family Law Reform 386

Re: W (a minor) Medical treatment: a court's jurisdiction (1992) 3 Weekly Law Report 758

Reed J (1992) Individualised nursing care: some implications. *J Clin Nurs* 1: 7–12

Reed P (1992a) An emerging paradigm for the investigation of spirituality in nursing. *Res Nurs Health* 15: 349–57

Rehm R S (2000) Family culture and chronic conditions. In: Ludder-Jackson P, Vessey JA, eds. *Primary Care of the Child with a chronic condition*, 3rd edn. Mosby, St Louis

Robertson J (1958) *Young Children in Hospital*. Tavistock Publications, London

Royal College of Nursing (2003) *Restraining, Holding Still and Containing Children and Young People*. RCN, London

Royal College of Nursing (2003a) *Child Protection—Every Nurse's Responsibility*. RCN, London

Royal College of Nursing (1994) *Standards of Care: Paediatric Nursing*, 2nd edn. RCN, Harrow

Sainsbury CPQ, Gray OP, Cleary J, *et al* (1986) Care by parents of their children in hospital. *Arch Dis Child* 61: 612–15

Santrock JW (1998) *Child Development*, 8th edn. McGraw-Hill, New York

Seden J (1998) The Spiritual Needs of Children. *Practice* 10(4): 57–67

Smith J, McSherry W (2003) The meaning of spirituality within the context of child development: a concept analysis. *J Adv Nurs* 45(3):1–8

Smith L, Coleman V, Bradshaw M (2002) Family-centred care: a practice continuum. In: Smith L, Coleman V, Bradshaw M, eds. *Family-Centred Care: Concepts, Theory and Practice*. Palgrave, Hampshire

Spencer GE (2000) Children's competency to consent: an ethical dilemma. *J Child Health Care* 4(3): 117–21

Steen S, Anderson B (1995) Ages and stages of spiritual development. *J Christian Nurs* 12(2): 6–11

Thompson C *et al* (2001) Research information in nurses' clinical decision-making: what is useful? *J Adv Nurs* 36(3): 376–88

Thornes R (1983) Parental access and family facilities in children's wards in England. *Br Med J* 287(2): 190–92

Vydelingum V (2000) South Asian patients' lived experience of acute care in an English hospital: a phenomenological study. *J Adv Nurs* 32(1): 100–107

Waters K, Easton N (1999) Individualised care: is it possible to plan and carry out? *J Adv Nurs* 29: 79–87

Webb B (1993) Trauma and tedium: an account of living on a children's ward. In: Walmsley J, Reynolds J, Shakespeare P, Wolf R, eds. *Health, Welfare and Practice: Reflecting on Roles and Relationships*. Sage, London: 184-89

Webb N, Hull D, Madeley R (1985) Care by parents in hospital. *Br Med J* **291**: 176–77

Webster A (2000). The facilitating role of the play specialist. *Paediatr Nurs* **12**(7): 24–27

Whiting L (1999) Caring for children of differing cultures. *J Child Health Care* **3**(4): 33–37

Wong DI, Perry SE (1998) *Maternal Child Nursing Care*. Mosby, Philadelphia

Zoucha R (2000) The keys to culturally sensitive care. *Am J Nurs* **100**(2): 24GG–24II

THREE

RECOGNISING AND MANAGING THE SERIOUSLY ILL CHILD

All healthcare staff working with children must be able to recognise and manage the seriously ill child. This is particularly important in the surgical environment, because:

- The administration of anaesthetic drugs induces unconsciousness, resulting in inadequate respiratory effort and a potential for airway obstruction

- Surgical and anaesthetic techniques may compromise the child's ability to maintain normal physiological controls post-operatively, such as a potential compromise to the airway, fluid and electrolyte imbalances, pain, haemorrhage and altered thermoregulation (Noble *et al*, 1997)

- Children admitted acutely, particularly following major trauma or where there is major loss or disruption to fluid distribution (such as intussusception), require rapid cardiopulmonary assessment and management to ensure survival.

This chapter will outline the anatomical and physiological differences between the child and adult that require consideration in relation to the peri-operative period, the knowledge required to recognise an acutely ill child, the principles of paediatric basic life-support and the principles of managing respiratory failure and shock.

3.1 Anatomical and physiological differences

Children have a low residual respiratory capacity, a high minute ventilation and cardiac output, a high metabolic rate and a large body surface area in relation to weight, therefore pathophysiological changes, such as hypoxia, hypercarbia, hypovolaemia and hypothermia can occur quickly. The major considerations in relation to anatomical and physiological differences between a child and adult in relation to peri-operative care are related to body size, airway management, fluid and electrolyte management and thermoregulation (Noble *et al*, 1997). These differences are most marked in the neonate and infant.

Body size

Body size is the most obvious difference across the age span. However, it is the proportional differences between height, weight and, particularly, surface area that are important (*figure 3.1a*) (Noble *et al*, 1997) because of the direct relationship to basal metabolic rate. Basal metabolic rate influences fluid and nutrition requirements, heat loss and drug uptake and clearance (Hazinski and Jenkins, 2002; Huether, 2002; Huether and Leo, 2002).

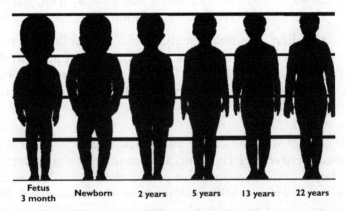

| Fetus 3 month | Newborn | 2 years | 5 years | 13 years | 22 years |

Figure 3.1a: Relative body proportions across the age span (adapted from Crouch and McClintic, 1976)

The selection of equipment, for example laryngoscopes, endotracheal tubes and face mask sizes, theatre instruments, positioning devices, tourniquets, sutures, and electrosurgical grounding pads, are all determined by size of the child (Noble *et al*, 1997).

Airway and respiratory system

A young child's airway differs markedly from that of an adult. A short neck, narrow nares, small pharynx, relatively large tongue in comparison to the rest of the oral cavity and the high position of the larynx, which pushes the tongue upwards towards the roof of the mouth, result in an increased risk of airway obstruction in the child (Noble *et al*, 1997). Children have narrow airways. The cricoid cartilage is the narrowest part of the airway, compared to the vocal cord in an adult; therefore the diameter of the endotracheal tube must fit through the cricoid ring (Noble *et al*, 1997). Any degree of oedema or secretion accumulation in a child's airway causes an exponentially greater reduction in diameter of the lumen compared to an adult (Froh, 2002). There is a concomitant increase in airway resistance resulting in an increased work rate of breathing (Chameides and Hazinski, 1997).

Infants up to six months of age are obligatory nasal breathers (Froh, 2002). The epiglottis is short, narrow, floppy and more 'U'-shaped; the vocal chords are shorter and more concave in comparison to an adult, making intubation and maintaining an airway more difficult. The thorax of the infant is small and the sternum is soft, the ribs are more pliable making the mechanical movement of the lungs more difficult and increasing the potential for paroxysmal movements rather than true lung expansion. The diaphragm has a much more important role to play in lung expansion in children (Froh, 2002).

The higher metabolic rate of children, and therefore oxygen consumption, results in any compromises to ventilation having a rapid effect on the ability to maintain adequate oxygenation (Froh, 2002). The average oxygen consumption of an infant is 6–8ml/kg/minute compared to 3–4 ml/kg/minute in adults (Chameides and Hazinski, 1997). In order to maintain this demand for oxygen, and the fact that the respiratory system is not fully developed until about eight years of age, means that the respiratory rate in children is much faster than adults (Froh, 2002). Although the respiratory drive, in terms of responding to hypercarbia, is present in the term newborn (McCance and Huether, 2002), the ability to handle stress is not as effective compared to older infants and children. Factors that have the potential to reduce respiratory drive in the newborn includes drugs, particularly anaesthetic agents and opioids, hypothermia and hypoglycemia.

Fluid and electrolytes

There are major differences between the child and adult in relation to the ability to maintain normal fluid and electrolytes (Noble *et al*, 1997). Firstly, although the circulating blood volume in children is approximately 75–80mls/kg, overall the total volume is small (Ratcliffe, 1998). Infants and children have a higher percentage of water content than adults, with the majority of this extra fluid lying within the extracellular fluid compartment. Children have a reduced ability to handle fluids and electrolytes, due to an immature renal system. The child is unable to withstand fluid imbalances compared to an adult, therefore requires a greater amount of free water to exchange electrolytes, particularly sodium (Huether, 2002). Dehydration, fluid excess, or changes in electrolyte concentrations can result in the child being unable to maintain a normal electrolyte balance and can have serious consequences, including death.

Management of fluids in the perioperative phase begins pre-operatively by ensuring the child is not fasted excessively (section 4.1). If the child is unable to tolerate oral fluids due to the underlying condition, an intravenous infusion must be sited. Intra-operatively, sufficient fluid replacement is necessary to cover the period the child has fasted and replace fluid losses which may have occurred during surgery. The type and amount of fluid administered must be based upon the child's weight, clinical needs, electrolyte results and potential expected losses. The type of fluids prescribed in children should reflect a child's inability to handle extreme concentrations of saline, dextrose and potassium. Normal maintenance fluids for infants and small children should contain a solution of 0.45 percent saline (Ratcliffe, 1998). Dextrose is necessary due to lack of fuel reserves in the infant and young child. The rate of administration of maintenance fluids should be calculated on body weight:

100ml/kg/day for the first 10 kg of the child's weight +

50ml/kg/day for the next 10 kg of the child's weight +
20ml/kg/day for the subsequent kg of the child's weight

(Ratcliffe 1998)

Cardiovascular system

Effective cardiac output is dependent upon the heart rate (beats per minute) and stroke volume (amount of blood ejected during each ventricular contraction), which is dependent upon venous return and the strength of myocardial contractions (Connor, 2002). With decreased age, there is less ability to increase the contractibility of the heart. Increases in cardiac output are primarily achieved by increasing the heart rate (Chameides and Hazinski, 1997). Normal blood pressure is maintained by having an adequate cardiac output and effective systemic vascular resistance (Chameides and Hazinski, 1997). In order to maintain an adequate blood pressure, necessary for tissue perfusion, a fall in cardiac output must be compensated for by vasoconstriction. Fortunately, children can maintain their blood pressure fairly well in the face of most insults. Therefore, a child who is hypotensive will already be in a state of circulatory collapse and requires immediate management (Chameides and Hazinski, 1997). Both bradycardia and prolonged tachycardia can result in inadequate cardiac output. Hypoxia in infants causes bradycardia (Connor, 2002) and is an ominous sign, usually indicating imminent arrest (Chameides and Hazinski, 1997).

Thermoregulation

Infants have a reduced ability to maintain a normal body temperature. Although they produce sufficient heat, they are unable to conserve heat because of an increased surface area, a thinner layer of insulating fat, and thinner dermis and epidermis, resulting in greater heat loss compared with an adult (Huether and Leo, 2002). Typical core body temperature is usually considered to be within the range of 36.2 to 37.7°C (McCance and Huether, 2002). However, body temperature is affected by a range of intrinsic and extrinsic factors (such as size, mass, age, sex, emotions, exercise, hormones) and displays a decrement from infancy to maturity (Smith, 1998).

Temperature extremes are not well tolerated in the infant; for example, in the critically ill infant, the physiological response to hypothermia will be to increase the metabolic rate, with a resultant increase in oxygen demands, which can further compromise respiratory and circulatory distress (Heath, 1998). Assisting the child to maintain normal body temperature in relation to the intra-operative period is discussed in section 4.2.

3.2　Recognising respiratory failure and shock

Recognising respiratory failure

Normal spontaneous respiration should occur with minimal effort and is usually a quiet process (Chameides and Hazinski, 1997). Respiratory rate is inversely related to age, reflecting neonates' and young infants' demand for oxygen, necessary to maintain rapid growth. Average respiratory rates relating to age are typically (Advanced Life Support Group, 2001):

Age	Respiratory rate (breaths per minute)
Newborn	40 – 60
< 1	30 – 40
2 – 5	25 – 30
5 – 12	20 – 25
> 12	15 – 20

These rates are guidelines; factors such as anxiety, exercise, fever, and pain will cause an increase in respiratory rates.

Respiratory failure will occur if there is inadequate respiration or oxygenation, usually a result of intrinsic disease of the respiratory system, airway obstruction or inadequate respiratory effort (Chameides and Hazinski, 1997). In general, respiratory failure is usually preceded by a period of respiratory distress, where the child attempts to maintain adequate oxygenation by increasing the rate and depth of breathing. Clinical observations are essential in order to recognise the child in respiratory distress and therefore at risk of respiratory failure and collapse

(Chameides and Hazinski, 1997). Over-reliance on blood gas analysis, which although it will indicate the severity of respiratory failure by determining the degree of hypoxia, hypercarbia and acidosis, can hinder the speed of managing the child in potential respiratory failure, unless blood sampling and analysis are immediately available (Chameides and Hazinski, 1997). A child in respiratory distress will usually present with:

- Alterations in respiratory rate
  - ○ Tachypneoa will be the initial response in an attempt to maintain oxygenation and a normal blood pH
  - ○ A slow and irregular respiratory rate in an acutely ill infant is an ominous sign and is usually the consequence of extreme fatigue
- Attempts to increased respiratory effort will result in visible signs, such as:
  - ○ Nasal flaring
  - ○ Intercostal, subcostal and suprasternal inspiratory recession
  - ○ Head bobbing
  - ○ Grunting
  - ○ Inspiratory stridor
  - ○ Prolonged expiration and expiratory wheeze
- Tachycardia
- Changes in skin colour and temperature will occur in response to vasoconstriction as blood is diverted from the extremities, in an attempt to increase oxygen supply to vital organs:
  - ○ Moderate hypoxia will cause pale or cyanosed mucous membranes, nail beds and extremities
  - ○ Severe hypoxia will cause central cyanosis, such as skin mottling over limbs and trunk
  - ○ Poor skin perfusion will cause cooling of the extremities

- ○ Differences between the core and peripheral temperatures will increase as respiratory distress increases
- ○ Capillary refill will decrease as skin perfusion decreases
- Poor cerebral perfusion will result in confusion and eventual loss of consciousness
- Children have reduced fatigue resistant muscle fibres, therefore tire easily.

Recognising shock

Shock is the term used to indicate a clinical state, where cardiovascular functioning is unable to deliver enough oxygen and metabolites to meet tissue demands, resulting in an accumulation of waste products (Chameides and Hazinski, 1997). Ultimately inadequate organ and tissue perfusion alters function and causes death. Shock is either classified in terms of aetiology (hypovolaemic, cardiogenic, septicaemic, neurogenic, anaphylactic) or on the effect of cardiac output and blood pressure (compensatory or decompensatory) (*Table 3.2a*). Although the classification of shock can be helpful in terms of definitive treatment, this tends to oversimplify the pathophysiological processes occurring, which are interrelated (Chameides and Hazinski, 1997). For example, the majority of children in shock, regardless of the cause, will have a degree of cardiovascular dysfunction. Furthermore, although respiratory failure and shock may begin as distinct clinical problems, the final stage for both, if untreated, is cardiopulmonary arrest.

Table 3.2a: Classification of shock (adapted from Ratcliffe, 1998, and Chameides and Hazinski, 1997)

Classification	Characteristics
Hypovolaemic shock	There is loss of fluid from the circulatory system; this could be due to direct blood loss or fluid losses, or more covertly due to mis-distribution of fluids.
Septicaemic shock	There is a systemic inflammatory response triggered by an invading micro-organism, which causes a complex immune amplification process. The key pathological process is extreme capillary leakage; the resultant hypovolaemia and hypotension compromise tissue oxygen delivery. There is also impaired ventricular contraction.
Cardiogenic shock	Collective term used to describe a range of cardiac conditions which result in inadequate left ventricular output. Ventricular output does not meet tissue demands.
Neurogenic shock	There is loss of sympathetic tone, for example, following spinal injury, which results in an inability to maintain the blood pressure.
Anaphylactic shock	Cell mediated immune response resulting in acute vasodilatation and capillary permeability. The result is a life-threatening fall in blood pressure.
Compensatory shock	The child presents with signs of inadequate organ perfusion, but blood pressure remains within normal limits.
Decompensatory shock	The child presents with signs of inadequate organ perfusion and a low blood pressure.

A child in shock will present with:

- Alterations in heart rate:
  - Tachycardia will be the initial response in an attempt to maintain oxygenation and a normal blood pH, although it must be noted that the neonate's response to hypoxia is usually bradycardia
  - Bradycardia ensues if tachycardia fails to maintain adequate tissue oxygenation, and is an ominous sign

- Alterations to systemic perfusion:
  - Discrepancy between central and peripheral pulse volumes
  - Changes in skin colour (mottling, pallor and cyanosis), cooling of the skin (initially a difference between the peripheral and core temperatures, but as shock continues, core temperature will fall)

- O Delayed capillary refill (greater than two seconds) (evaluating capillary refill necessitates lifting the limb to the level of the heart to ensure arteriole capillaries are being assessed)
- O Poor skin turgor
- Alterations in blood pressure:
  - O Normal blood pressure will be maintained, despite a fall in cardiac output and systemic vascular resistance, if compensatory vasoconstriction occurs
  - O When compensatory mechanisms fail, hypotension occurs and is a late, often sudden and ominous sign of cardiovascular insufficiency
- End organ perfusion failure:
  - O Hypoperfusion of the brain results in confusion, irritability, failure to recognise parents and lethargy. Cerebral oedema with more obvious neurological signs, such as unconsciousness, failure to respond to painful stimuli, seizures, dilated unreactive pupils, and loss of muscular tone, is an indication of severe hypoxia
  - O Poor renal perfusion will occur as a result of hypovolaemia; a reduced urine output (normal being 1–2 ml/kg per hour) will indicate the degree of hypovolaemia
- Depressed fontanel
- Increased respirations.

Typical values for heart rate and blood pressure are (Advanced Life Support Group, 2001):

Age	Heart rate (beats per minute)
Newborn	100 – 180
< 1	110 – 160
2 – 5	95 – 140
5 – 12	80 – 120
> 12	60 – 100

Age	Systemic blood pressure (mmHg)
Newborn	60 – 80
< 1	70 – 90
2 – 5	80 – 100
5 – 12	90 – 110
> 12	100 – 120

Rapid cardiopulmonary assessment of seriously ill child

It is essential that healthcare professionals can recognise potential respiratory distress and shock in children, and impending cardiopulmonary arrest (Chameides and Hazinski, 1997). This requires a systematic and rapid approach to assessing the child. The assessment should take no longer than one minute and aim to determine if the child:

- Is stable

- Has a potential for respiratory failure or shock

- Is in definite respiratory failure or shock

- Is in cardiopulmonary failure.

The rapid cardiopulmonary assessment includes assessment of (Chameides and Hazinski, 1997):

- The airway
  - o Maintaining independently
  - o Requir ingassistance
- Breathing
  - o Rate
  - o Mechanics, such as presence of recession, grunting, nasal flaring and use of accessory muscles
  - o Air entry, such as degree of chest expansion and paradoxical chest movements, quality of breaths' sounds, presence of stridor and wheezing
- Circulation
  - o Heart rate
  - o Blood pressure

- ○ Presence/absence of peripheral pulses
- ○ Estimation of skin perfusion such as colour, temperature
- ○ Capillary refill time
- Disability
  - ○ Level of consciousness (AVPU scale—Alert, responds to Voice, responds to Pain, Unconscious)
  - ○ Pupil reactions
  - ○ Muscle tone
  - ○ Posture
  - ○ Convulsions.

Once the rapid assessment has been conducted and the level of support the child requires has been identified, appropriate interventions and investigations, such as blood sampling and capillary glucose monitoring, can begin. If at any time during the rapid assessment the child becomes unresponsive, the assessment should be stopped and basic life support commenced.

A severely ill child will be an overwhelming and traumatic experience for the family, who will need support and accurate and timely information.

3.3 Basic life support

Basic life support (BLS) is comprised of an initial assessment, airway maintenance, rescue breathing and chest compressions (Resuscitation Council UK, 2000). Modern cardio-pulmonary resuscitation did not develop until the 1960s. Publication of the 2000 guidelines is the first truly international approach to BLS (Resuscitation Council UK, 2000). They represent a unified approach to BLS through the work of the European Resuscitation Council, International Liaison Committee on Resuscitation, and Resuscitation Council UK and reflect the best available evidence in relation to life support techniques. Although there is a common approach to BLS, it must be noted that each of the councils' publications may differ slightly, particularly in relation to terminology, which reflects local custom and practices. The following description of basic life support for children reflects the guidance set out by the Resuscitation Council UK (2000), which incorporated the American Heart Association (2000) and the European Resuscitation (1998) guidelines. The guidelines can be utilised by non-healthcare professionals and are therefore relevant for educating carers, if their child's condition necessitates learning BLS skills. The guidelines relating to healthcare professionals are described here. All staff should be competent in performing BLS.

Definitions

The Resuscitation Council UK (2000) define:

- BLS as the maintenance of the airway while providing support for breathing and the circulatory system without the assistance of equipment

- An infant as under one year of age, a young child is one to eight years

- A child over eight years of age is treated as young child, but *may* require 'adult' techniques to attain adequate circulation.

Epidemiology

The causes of cardio-respiratory arrest in children are different from adults because:

- The hearts of infants and young children are usually healthy

- Primary cardiac arrest is rare in children

- In the infant, respiratory arrest is the more common scenario and usually follows deterioration of respiratory function

- In the older infant and child, cardio-respiratory arrest is commonly due to progression of respiratory failure or following shock or neurological dysfunction

- Hypoxia is usually severe before the heart ceases to function.

Outcome

In children, respiratory arrest precedes cardiac arrest in most cases. Cardiac arrest has a poor outcome because:

- Respiratory arrest precedes asystole, therefore profound hypoxia and hypercarbia have already occurred prior to cardiac arrest

- There is often poor neurological function (even if BLS has been successful) following cardiac arrest due to the heart being able to function under severe hypoxia compared with the brain and other vital organs.

It is vital that a seriously ill child is recognised in order to instigate early management and prevent cardio-pulmonary arrest occurring. If a child arrests, the aim is to maintain ventilation and begin BLS.

Sequence of action when performing BLS

Figure 3.3a outlines the sequence of actions when performing BLS, and the specific manoeuvres for infant, child and adolescent. This should be a refresher for all staff caring for children and should complement annual mandatory training.

Assessment phase for each procedure should
take no more than 10 seconds

**ENSURE SAFETY OF RESCUER AND
CHILD: APPROACH WITH CARE**

CHECK THE CHILD'S RESPONSIVENESS

**Ask loudly if child alright
Stimulate by gently shaking the child (unless
cervical injury suspected)**

If responsive do not change position
of child
unless in danger
Activate emergency call system
Reassess regularly

If not responsive evaluate:
Activate emergency call system
If possible, leave child in position
you find them
Assess: Airway Breathing,
Circulation

Airway

Open child's airway using chin-lift (Figure 3.3b)
Place hand on forehead and lift head back
With the other hand, place fingers on and lift the chin to
open airway; avoid pressing on soft tissue
If neck injury is suspected, use jaw-thrust (Figure 3.3c)
Check and remove any obvious obstructions (but do not
use a blind finger sweep to check airway is clear)

If breathing, place on side,
get help, continue monitoring
and maintain airway

If not breathing,
proceed
as below

Figure 3.3a Sequences of actions when performing BLS (Resuscitation
Council UK 2000)

Table 3.3a: Sequences of actions when performing BLS (Resuscitation Council UK 2000)

Action	Infant	Young Child	Older Child
Breathing	Carefully remove any obstructions Give up to five rescue breaths of which two must be effective in ensuring the chest rises and falls **Rescue breaths** Maintain airway (chin lift) Take a breath, cover the infant's nose and mouth with your mouth ensuring a good seal Blow steadily into infant's nose and mouth for 1–1.5 seconds, to ensure chest rises Observe chest falling, take another breath and repeat	Carefully remove any obstructions Give up to five rescue breaths of which two must be effective in ensuring the chest rises and falls **Rescue breaths** Maintain airway (chin lift) Close the child's nose by pinching the soft part of nose, with the index finger and thumb of the hand on the forehead Take a breath, cover child's mouth with your mouth ensuring a good seal Blow steadily into child's mouth for 1–1.5 seconds, to ensure chest rises Observe chest falling, take another breath and repeat	Carefully remove any obstructions Give up to five rescue breaths of which two must be effective in ensuring the chest rise and falls **Rescue breaths** Maintain airway (chin lift) Close the child's nose by pinching the soft part of nose, with the index finger and thumb of the hand on the forehead Take a breath, cover child's mouth with your mouth ensuring a good seal Blow steadily into child's mouth for 1–1.5 seconds, to ensure chest rises Observe chest falling, take another breath and repeat
Circulation	Assess for signs of circulation such as no movements, unresponsive, not breathing and inadequate pulse (by feeling for the brachial pulse) If you are confident there is no circulatory collapse continue rescue breathing and regular circulatory assessment If there are no signs of circulation or the pulse is inadequate to maintain circulation (i.e. below 60 beats per minute) commence chest compressions Locate and place two fingers on the sternum (one finger breadth below an imaginary line joining the infant's nipples) Depress the sternum one third of infant's chest, allow chest to rise by releasing the pressure and repeat five times	Assess for signs of circulation such as no movements, unresponsive, not breathing and inadequate pulse (by feeling for carotid pulse) If you are confident there is no circulatory collapse continue rescue breathing and regular circulatory assessment If there are no signs of circulation or the pulse is inadequate to maintain circulation (i.e. below 60 beats per minute) commence chest compressions Locate and place the heel of one hand on the sternum (one finger breadth above the xiphisternum) Positioned vertically above the child depress the sternum one third of child's chest, allow chest to rise by releasing the pressure and repeat five times	Assess for signs of circulation such as no movements, unresponsive, not breathing and inadequate pulse (by feeling for carotid pulse) If you are confident there is no circulatory collapse continue rescue breathing and regular circulatory assessment If there are no signs of circulation or the pulse is inadequate to maintain circulation (i.e. below 60 beats per minute) commence chest compressions Locate and place the heel of two hands, with the fingers interlocked and raised to avoid finger pressure, on the sternum (one finger breadth above the xiphisternum) Positioned vertically above the child depress the sternum one third of child's chest, allow chest to rise by releasing the pressure and repeat 15 times

Continuation of BLS	Combine chest compressions and breaths at a ratio of 5:1
	Continue until:
	  Signs of life appear (spontaneous respirations and pulse)
	  Help arrives
	  You become exhausted		

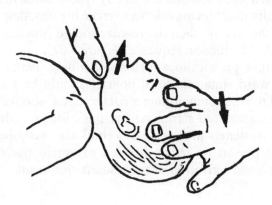

Figure 3.3b: Chin lift

A child who is unconscious, but maintaining his/her own airway should be placed in the recovery position (unless cervical injury is suspected) *(Figure 3.3d)* to prevent the tongue from falling back and obstructing the airway. It may be necessary to modify techniques in the infant and small child, such as providing a support placed in hollow of the back to maintain the position. However, the principles of the recovery position, placing in a true lateral position, allowing the airway to remain open to facilitate drainage of secretions and easy access of airway should be maintained (Resuscitation Council UK, 2000).

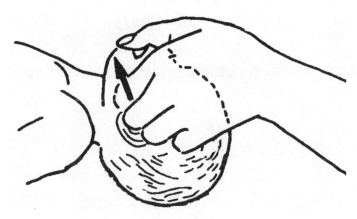

Figure 3.3c: Jaw thrust

If there is a suspicion that the airway is obstructed because there is difficulty in achieving effective rescue breaths, despite re-positioning the airway, then the rescuer should proceed to the foreign body obstruction sequence (*Figure 3.3e*).

Other practicalities include obtaining assistance. In the clinical ward situation, local policies should be followed and adhered to when summoning assistance. Staff should be familiar with emergency call alarm systems. Basic life procedures should begin immediately in the case of a child who has collapsed, with the next person to arrive directed to obtain the appropriate assistance and activation of the resuscitation team.

3.4 Managing respiratory failure and shock

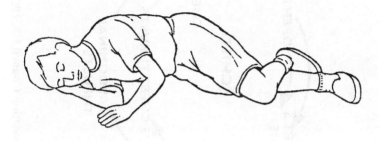

Figure 3.3d: Recovery position

Managing respiratory failure

The aims of care are to anticipate problems and support or replace respiratory functions that are compromised or lost (Chameides and Hazinski, 1997). The child in respiratory distress will often find a position that is comfortable and causes the least distress; therefore, unless the airway is compromised he/she should not be moved. For a child who has a compromised airway or is unconscious/unresponsive but breathing, maintaining a patent airway is a vital. In the absence of airway adjuncts, this can be achieved using the chin lift, jaw thrust or placing the child in the recovery position (*Figures 3.3b, c, d*). Airway adjuncts include:

- *Oropharyngeal (Geudel) airway:* can be used in conjunction with chin lift/jaw thrust, to assist in maintaining the airway in an unconscious child by preventing the tongue falling backwards. The airway size (00, 0, 1, 2, 3) can be estimated by placing the flange at the centre of the mouth and placing the airway towards the ear lobe: the correct length would be just to the angle of the jaw. An incorrect size will further compromise the airway; if too large it will

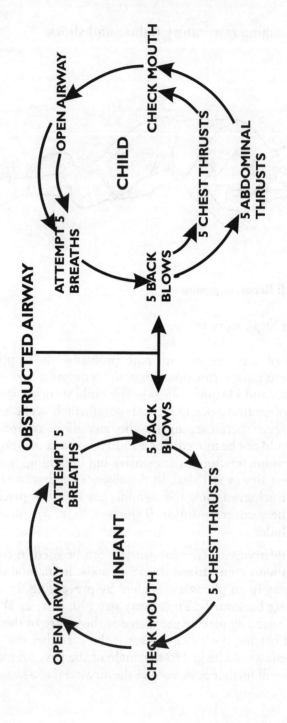

Figure 3.3e: Sequence of actions for managing an obstructed airway (Resuscitation Council UK 2000)

obstruct the larynx, and if too small it will push the tongue back obstructing the pharynx. In a child and adult, it is easier to insert the airway by holding the flange with the tip of the airway pointing upwards and rotating the airway to pass over the tongue, which is held in place by a tongue depressor. In an infant with a relatively small mouth, large tongue and softer palate, this technique may cause trauma, therefore the airway should be inserted directly, while ensuring it is over the tongue

- *Nasopharyngeal airway:* these latex airways are more flexible and inserted through a nostril, and are tolerated better in responsive patients. However, the small internal diameter easily blocks with secretions.

(Chameides and Hazinski, 1997)

Oropharyngeal, nasopharyngeal or tracheal suctioning of secretions, blood or vomitus may be required to maintain a clear airway. However, suctioning is not without risks including hypoxemia, cardiac dysrythmias, trauma, bleeding and infection (Hackeling *et al*, 1998; Kapadia *et al*, 2000). These risk factors are compounded by the poor knowledge of many nurses relating to suctioning procedures (Day *et al*, 2001; 2002). Principles of suction- ing in an acutely ill child include:

- Assess the child for the need for suctioning, including the presence of secretions and chest auscultation

- Adequate preparation of the child and family

- Pre-oxygenate

- Maintaining a sterile procedure

- For tracheostomy or tracheal suctioning, the external diameter of catheter should not exceed one half the diameter of the tube

- Catheters should be flexible and cause minimal trauma

- Minimal negative pressure, between 80–150mmHg, should be applied only on withdrawal of the catheter for a maximum of 10–15 seconds.

(Day *et al*, 2001; Wood, 1998)

Respiratory distress, shock and trauma will all compromise the ability to provide tissues with sufficient oxygen; therefore oxygen therapy is a high priority in the overall management of the seriously ill child. The techniques used to administer oxygen must meet the clinical needs of the child. Oxygen delivery systems include:

- *Simple face masks,* available in different sizes, should be available in all areas that care for children and will deliver oxygen between 35–60 percent when flow rates are set between 6–10 litres/minute

- *Partial rebreathable masks* have a reservoir and can deliver oxygen at between 50–60 percent when flow rates are set between 10–12 litres/minute

- *Non-rebreathable bags* have a reservoir and valve, which ensures that the oxygen delivered is direct from the source and not mixed with environmental or expired air; therefore high delivery rates of oxygen between 95–100 percent when flow rates are set between 10–12 litres/minute can be achieved

- *Oxygen tents, hood head boxes* are available, which provide a contained environment into which oxygen can be delivered. They are often suitable for the infant who cannot tolerate a face mask. However, it is difficult to predict and maintain the level of oxygen within these systems. An oxygen analyser will be necessary to monitor oxygen levels within the system

- *Nasal cannulae* are prongs inserted into the nostrils and can be used to deliver oxygen via the nasopharynx. However, these are usually only tolerated by infants and only suitable when low concentrations of oxygen are required because humidification is not possible, flow rates above 4 litres/minute are irritant to the nasopharynx and precise delivery rates of oxygen are difficult to achieve.

(Chameides and Hazinski, 1997; Chandler, 2001)

If the child is responding well to oxygen therapy and the rapid assessment has been completed, as soon as practicably possible oxygen therapy should include humidification and warming, unless there is a clear indication that the use of oxygen is a short-term measure (Chandler, 2001). For example, in the immediate post-operative period, oxygen is usually administered while there is potential for continued effects of anaesthetic drugs, which may render the child's respiratory rate and effort being insufficient to maintain adequate oxygen levels.

Pulse oximetry is an effective and frequently used method of monitoring oxygen saturation levels in children, for example in the immediate post-operative period, during acute respiratory illness and, more recently, to aid in the assessment of conditions such as sleep-disordered breathing (Chandler, 2000; Urschitz *et al*, 2003). All children receiving oxygen therapy should have their oxygen saturation levels monitored (Chandler, 2001). A pulse oximeter measures arterial blood oxygen saturation (SpO_2) by estimating the oxygen saturation of haemoglobin, when two light-emitting diodes and a photosensitive detector are placed across a tissue bed, typically across a finger or toe (Chameides and Hazinski, 1997; Chandler, 2000). The sensitivity of recordings is dependent upon many factors, including the type of monitor. New generation monitors have a greater capacity to compensate for artifacts, such as motion and poor circulation (Bohnhorst *et al*, 2000). Few studies that have produced reliable data for normal reference values for SpO_2 levels in children. Overnight SpO_2 levels in children are typically around 98 percent, with the median range between 94 and 100 percent (Urschitz *et al*, 2003). In the acutely ill child, pulse oximetry is invaluable in that it provides a continuous method of evaluating arterial oxygen saturation (Chameides and Hazinski, 1997). There are limitations to the use of pulse oximetry, namely, although oxygenation is monitored, the effectiveness of respirations (carbon dioxide elimination) is not measured; recordings are dependent upon a pulsatile blood flow and will not provide reliable, therefore useful, information on a child in shock or with poor peripheral perfusion (Chameides and Hazinski, 1997).

It will be necessary in the case of the non-breathing child, and in the best interests of a child in severe respiratory distress, to ventilate the child. It is not within the scope of this text to provide details of ventilatory support in children. However, in the intra-operative period, healthcare professionals may require the skills, particularly if working in an extended role within anaesthesia, to be competent in bag-valve mask ventilation. Principles of bag-mask ventilation:

- The system consists of a face mask which must be able to provide a good seal over the child's nose and mouth, without applying pressure to the eyes, an appropriate sized compressible bag (500ml for an infant, 1000—1500ml for a child over one year of age), an oxygen connection point, a pop-off valve (this prevents over-inflation of the lungs once lung resistance occurs) and an air entry/reservoir point

- For successful ventilation there must be an unobstructed airway, a tight face mask seal and compression of the bag at a rate of 20 cycles per minute

- Unless connected to oxygen, then environmental air will be delivered

- Consider passing a naso-gastric tube to deflate the stomach of gases that may accumulate up during ventilation techniques.

Managing shock and haemorrhage

Although shock can have several aetiologies (*Table 3.2a*), the most common cause worldwide is hypovolaemia (Chameides and Hazinski, 1997). Hypovolaemia is a characteristic of all forms of shock because, independent of the cause, as shock progresses there is always a resultant vasodilatation, increased capillary permeability and plasma loss into the interstitial fluid spaces. The initial aim of care in all forms of shock is to restore circulatory volume (Ratcliffe 1998). The definitive management of the different types of shock is outlined in *Table 3.4a*. The principles for managing shock are:

- Rapid assessment of airway, breathing and circulation (section 3.1)

- Face mask oxygen

- Rapid venous access to be achieved within two minutes; if it is not possible to insert a wide-bore, peripheral vascular catheter then an intraosseous needle must be inserted (the preferred site being the tibial tuberosity)

- Fluid resuscitation necessitates rapid infusion of volume expanders at a rate of 20ml/kg over 20 minutes, followed by reassessment and further fluid boluses as necessary

- The ideal fluid in initial management of shock is either an isotonic crystalloid solution, such as 0.9 percent saline or a colloid solution such as 4.5 percent albumin. Saline has the advantage of being readily available, but results in a transient expansion of circulating fluid, therefore large quantities are necessary. Colloids remain in the intravascular compartment longer, but are more likely to cause sensitivity reactions

- Large volumes of dextrose-containing fluids should *not* be given because a resultant hyperglycemia causes an osmotic diuresis, which effectively causes fluid to be withdrawn from the circulatory system, exacerbating the hypovolaemia and causing hypokalaemia

- A child who is hypoglycaemic (determined by blood glucose levels) should receive a bolus of high concentration glucose (for example 10–20mls/kg of 5 percent dextrose)

- Insertion of a urinary catheter and measurement of urine output.

(Ratcliffe, 1998; Chameides and Hazinski, 1997)

If the signs and symptoms of shock are detected early and the child is managed effectively, stabilisation occurs fairly rapidly. The child will need regular reassessment and close monitoring. Subsequent fluid management will be based upon the clinical circumstances and underlying condition of the child. A child who does not respond to fluid resuscitation, for example peripheral circulation does not improve, blood pressure and pulse are labile and there is no urine output (Ratcliffe, 1998), will require more intensive management. The child will require the skills of a dedicated paediatric intensive care team and management, including ventilatory and inotropic support.

Table 3.4a: Definitive management of shock based upon aetiology (adapted from Ratcliffe, 1998)

Aetiology	Management
Hypovolaemic shock	Fluid resuscitation In severe dehydration and children who have not responded to initial management, transfer to paediatric intensive care for potential elective ventilation and inotropic support
Septicaemic shock	Fluid resuscitation Aim is to achieve adequate cardiovascular parameters, which will require repeated colloid infusion Antibiotic therapy In severe cases and children who have not responded to initial management, transfer to paediatric intensive care for potential elective ventilation and inotropic support
Cardiogenic shock	Fluid resuscitation Need to identify the cause and evaluate rhythm, and treat accordingly
Neurogenic shock	Fluid resuscitation A vasopressor infusion (nor-adrenaline) to support the blood pressure
Anaphylactic shock	Fluid resuscitation Rapid infusions of adrenaline, hydrocortisone and chlorpheniramine

Haemorrhage is a potential complication of surgery (Watcha, 2000). Therefore, the early detecting of haemorrhage is an essential component of post-operative care, and includes

- Careful observations of wound site, dressing and drains if present, for excessive oozing and fluid loss

- Cardiovascular monitoring (pulse, blood pressure, colour), observation of respiratory rate and effort

- Observations specific to the surgical procedure, for example excessive swallowing in oral surgery.

Blood losses of over 15 percent of the total circulatory volume will result in detectable signs of circulatory failure; namely, tachycardia, decreased peripheral pulses, delayed capillary refill and cool extremities (Chameides and Hazinski, 1997). Hypotension will be a late sign and probably not occur until blood losses are within the region of 20–30 percent of total circulatory volume. If there is any indication that a significant bleed has occurred and the child is in shock, then rapid cardiovascular assessment is required. Where possible external pressure to the wound site should be applied, oxygen should be administered and resuscitation fluid management commenced. Blood transfusion will be paramount because, although resuscitation fluids will help in restoration of the intravascular volume, loss of haemoglobin will severely reduce the ability to maintain tissue oxygenation and blood clotting factors will become depleted. In all but minor haemorrhages, surgical intervention will be necessary to control the bleeding.

References

Advanced Life Support Group (2001) *Advanced Paediatric Life Support: The Practical Approach,* 3rd edn. BMJ Publications, London

American Heart Association in Collaboration with the International Liaison Committee on Resuscitation (2000) Guidelines 2000 for cardiopulmonary resuscitation and emergency cardiovascular care. An international consensus on science. *Resuscitation* **46**: 1–448

Bohnhorst B, Peter CS, Poets CF (2000) Pulse oximeter's reliability in detecting hypoxemia and bradycardia: a comparrison between conventional and two new generation oximeters. *Crit Care Med* **28**: 1565–68

Chameides L, Hazinski MF (1997) *Pediatric Advanced Life Support.* American Heart Association, Texas

Chandler T (2001) Oxygen administration. *Paediatr Nurs* **13**(8): 37–42

Chandler T (2000) Oxygen saturation monitoring. *Paediatr Nurs* **12**(8): 37–42

Connor JA (2002) Alterations in cardiovascular function in children. In: McCance KL, Huether SE, eds. *Pathophysiology: The Biological Basis for Disease in Adults and Children,* 4th edn. Mosby, St Louis

Crouch JE, McClintic JR (1976) Human anatomy and physiology, 2nd edn. John Wiley and Sons Inc. New York

Day T, Farnell S, Haynes S *et al* (2002) Tracheal suctioning: an exploration of nurses' knowledge and competence in acute and high dependency ward areas. *J Adv Nurs* **39**(1): 35–45

Day T, Wainright S, Wilson-Barnett J (2001) An evaluation of a teaching intervention to improve the practice of endotracheal suctioning in intensive care units. *J Clin Nurs* **10**: 682–96

European Resuscitation Council (1998) Paediatric basic life support. *Resuscitation* **37**: 97–100

Froh DF (2002) Alterations of pulmonary function in children. In: McCance KL, Huether SE, eds. *Pathophysiology: The Biological Basis for Disease in Adults and Children,* 4th edn. Mosby, St Louis

Hackeling T, Triana R, John O *et al* (1998) Emergency care of patients with tracheostomies: a seven year review. *Am J Emerg Med* **16**: 681–85

Hazinski MF, Jenkins ME (2002) Shock, multiple organ dysfunction syndrome and burns in children. In: McCance KL, Huether SE, eds. *Pathophysiology: the Biological Basis for Disease in Adults and Children*, 4th edn. Mosby, St Louis

Heath S (1998) *Perioperative Care of the Child.* Mark Allen Publishing Ltd, Salisbury

Huether SE (2002) Alterations of renal dysfunction and urinary tract function in children. *Pathophysiology*: *The Biological Basis for Disease in Adults and Children*, 4th edn. Mosby, St Louis

Huether SE, Leo J (2002) Pain, temperature regulation, sleep and sensory function. *Pathophysiology*: *The Biological Basis for Disease in Adults and Children*, 4th edn. Mosby, St Louis

Kapadia FN, Bajan KB, Rajie KV (2000) Airway accidents in intubated intensive acre unit patients: an epidemiological study. *Crit Care Med* **28**: 659–64

McCance KL, Huether SE (2002) *Pathophysiology*: *The Biological Basis for Disease in Adults and Children*, 4th edn. Mosby, St Louis

Noble RR, Micheli AJ, Hensley MA *et al* (1997) Perioperative considerations for the pediatric patient: a developmental approach. *Nurs Clin N Am* **32**(10): 1–16

Ratcliffe JM (1998) Recognition and management of shock. *Curr Paediatrics* **8**: 1–5

Resuscitation Council UK (2000) *Resuscitation Guidelines 2000.* Resuscitation Council Publications, London

Smith J (1998) Are electronic thermometry techniques suitable alternatives to traditional mercury in glass thermometry techniques in the paediatric setting? *J Adv Nurs* **28**(5): 1030–39

Urschitz MS, Wolff J, Einem V *et al* (2003) Reference values for nocturnal home pulse oximetry during sleep in primary school children. *Chest* **121**(1): 96–101

Watcha M (2000) The immediate recovery period. In: Sumner E, Hatch DJ, eds. *Paediatric Anaesthesia*, 2nd edn. Arnold, London

Wood CJ (1998) Endotracheal suctioning: a literature review. *Intens Critic Care Nurs* **14**: 124–36

Further information

www.resus.org.uk

FOUR

PERIOPERATIVE NURSING CARE

Surgery and anaesthesia disrupt normal functioning, homeostatic mechanisms and are potentially life-threatening. The main goal of care must be aimed at minimising potential complications by ensuring the child and family are prepared appropriately and safely for surgery, and ensuring anaesthetic and recovery needs are met. In addition to ensuring the overall goals are achieved, the nurse should promote care that is patient-focused, and provide continuity before, during and after surgery (Cowan, 1998). Although interlinked, perioperative care is usually divided into three general phases, pre-, intra- and post-operative care (Leinonen and Leino-Kilpi, 1999), and will form the sections within this chapter.

The section relating to pre-operative care will focus upon the physical preparation of the child prior to surgery. These principles can be applied to the child admitted for both elective surgery and in an emergency. Issues crucial to pre-operative care, such as obtaining consent, family-centred care and the psychological preparation of the child and family for surgery, will not be revisited, as they are covered extensively elsewhere. The intra-operative section will focus upon the assessment and management of the child within the theatre environment in the broadest sense and will not provide explicit details of procedures and practices essential to effective management of care within the theatre environment. Practical aspects of care, such as airway management, fluid management, and the management of shock and haemorrhage, are covered in *Chapter 3*. The focus of the section relating to post-operative care will be related to maintaining the immediate physical safety of the child, detecting the potential complications of surgery and providing support for the child and family. Other aspects of post-operative care, such as the assessment and management of pain, wound care, discharge planning and ongoing community care are discussed within designated chapters.

4.1 Pre-operative care

Pre-operative care can be divided into three general areas: the psychological preparation of the child and family, optimising the health of the child prior to surgery and ensuring the physical safety of the child (Heath, 1998). The psychological preparation of children prior to surgery is discussed in *Chapter 7*.

Optimising the health of the child prior to surgery

The aim of pre-operative assessment is to ensure the child is in optimal health prior to anaesthesia and surgery (Heath, 1998). The assessment is a multidisciplinary approach and, although primarily involving the surgeon, the anaesthetist and nursing staff, can involve all members of the multidisciplinary team, depending upon the child's individual needs. The health assessment should include:

- An assessment of the child's current condition and the need for surgery

- Screening for the presence of unknown underlying abnormalities, which have the potential to influence the outcome of anaesthesia

- Effective planning to manage existing diseases, such as diabetes mellitus

- Identification of the child and parents' understanding of the surgery and any health education needs

- Identification of any psychological and social circumstances, which may have an impact upon the care needs of the child and family.

Health assessments involve a detailed medical and anaesthetic assessment and, although these assessments have been traditionally the remit of the surgeon and anaesthetist respectively, this is no longer the case. The transfer of traditional roles from doctors to nurses is a recent occurrence within the UK compared to countries such as the USA. Changes in practice have been driven primarily by the medical professional bodies and government policies, which have been critical of the repetitive and routine nature of much of the doctors' work and the need to reduce junior doctors hours (Department of Health, 1993; National Health Service Management Executive, 1991). The expansion of nursing responsibilities, as outlined in the Scope of Professional Practice (United Kingdom Central Council, 1992), paved the way for less demarcation between traditional doctor/nurse roles. The overall nursing response has been mixed, primarily because of the assumption that nurses will automatically undertake new tasks. However, there are potential benefits for the child and family including the delivery of seamless care and a potential reduction in the number of healthcare professionals the child and family encounter (Rushforth and Glasper, 1999). Unfortunately, there are inherent difficulties in changing practice when no evidence exists to support the effectiveness of the change. In addition, and despite strong drivers for change, it is paramount that the safety of the child and the quality of care are ensured. Therefore changes to care delivery must be effectively monitored. There appears to be only one randomised control trial of medical versus nurse-led clerking for children undergoing surgery within the UK (Rushforth *et al*, 2000; 2000a). Although, Rushforth *et al*'s research was a pilot study, with insufficient numbers to make generalisations, the results indicated that nurses may have superior skills in history-taking when compared with senior house officers. The nurses within the study performed better at identifying abnormalities, such as possible transfusion reactions, penicillin allergies, cardiac problems and asthma-related problems, which have perioperative implications. In addition, and despite pre-study anticipations, nurses were not over-cautious, with neither group wrongly identifying non-existent problems.

Whether nurse or medically-led, the pre-operative health assessment has two interrelated components; namely, history-taking and physical assessment (Rushforth *et al*, 2000a). The history should include a description of the current condition and its effects, current treatments (including complementary therapies) and medications, past medical history and ongoing health problems, previous anaesthetic history and complications, and identification of any known allergies (American Society of Anesthetists, 2002). For patients with high severity of disease classification, the assessment should be undertaken on the day prior to surgery. As a minimum, the physical examination should include an assessment of the airway, heart and lungs, and measurement and documentation of vital signs (American Society of Anesthetists, 2002). One of the major dilemmas for anaesthesiology in children is the decision relating to anaesthetising children who present with an upper respiratory infection (URI) (Brown *et al*, 2000; Tait *et al*, 2001). The presence of URI is associated with increased intra-operative complications, such as bronchospasm, laryngospasm and oxygen desaturation (Brown *et al*, 2000). Tait *et al*'s (2001) study suggests that the majority of children with an URI can undergo anaesthesia, because any complications that occur do not have any long-term effects. However, consideration needs to be given to the whole clinical picture, including the presence of a productive cough, fever, history of respiratory disease, such as asthma, presence of a wheeze and general malaise (Brown *et al*, 2000; Tait *et al*, 2001).

Traditionally, the physical assessment has included the routine ordering of pre-operative investigations, such as chest X-ray, electrocardiogram, blood samples and urinalysis (Munro *et al*, 1997). However, the majority of these tests are unnecessary, particularly if there are no anticipated complications, no anticipated blood loss and the surgery is of short duration. Therefore investigations should only be requested in the presence of a specific clinical condition or defined risks due to the nature of the surgical procedure (American Society of Anesthetists, 2002; Munro *et al*, 1997). Furthermore as the small percentage of abnormalities detected rarely, if ever, changes the management of the patient, the value and cost-effectiveness of undertaking these tests must be questioned (Munro *et al*, 1997). The American Society of Anesthesiologists Task Force on Pre-anesthesia Evaluation (American Society of Anesthetists, 2002) and the UK Health Technology Assessment

Programme (Munro *et al*, 1997) have both provided a comprehensive review of the evidence relating to the value of pre-operative testing and criteria for selecting an investigation in relation to patient characteristics. It is vital that the rationale for pre-operative investigations is clear, in order to avoid unnecessary procedures for the child.

In addition to coordinating the assessment process, the nurse will need to undertake a comprehensive nursing assessment. Unfortunately, repeated assessments by various professionals can become very tedious for the child and family. The increased use of common documentation (Brunt *et al*, 1999) and integrated care pathways (Currie and Harvey, 1997; Norris, 1998) has the potential for greater co-ordination in the assessment, treatment and evaluation of care across professional boundaries. However, there is a danger that a medical model of care will dominate, where patients are compartmentalised into body systems relating to specific health disorders (Lowe, 1998). Casey (1988) suggests that the purpose of a nursing assessment is to establish:

- Family care that the child usually requires
- Current condition of the child both physical and psychologically
- Nursing care the child requires in relation to both current diagnosis and general health needs
- Ability of the child and family to participate in care required.

In practice, the assessment is usually carried out through the application of a specific nursing model that guides the delivery of care through assessment, planning, implementation and evaluation, collectively referred to as the nursing process (Heath, 1998). Probably the most widely utilised nursing model within the UK is Roper, Logan and Tierney's Activities of Living Model (Tierney, 1998). The model is based upon the concept that an individual's ability to maintain the 12 activities of living (basic human needs) depends upon biological, psychological, sociocultural, environmental, and politicoeconomic factors (Roper *et al*, 1996; 1980). *Figure 4.1a* provides an overview of the model. The model is not without criticisms (Tierney, 1998), such as being biased towards physical aspects of care and overtly problem-orientated, therefore its application is more geared toward acute hospital-based care. There have been some attempts to develop nursing models specifically for the child and family (Happs, 1994), and include Partnership Model of Paediatric Nursing (Casey, 1988), Parent-Child Interaction Model (Baker *et al*, 1989) and the Nottingham Model (Smith, 1995).

Nurses working with the child and family will probably be most familiar with Casey's (1988) partnership model. It is based on the premise that 'the care of children, sick or well, is best carried out by their families with varying degrees of assistance from members of a suitably qualified healthcare team whenever possible' (Casey, 1988: 9). However, the model does not provide a framework, such as the activities of living, from which an assessment can be made (*Figure 4.1b*). This was not an omission, but a conscious decision by Casey (1988), who did not wish to place constraints upon nurses working with children with diverse needs and within a variety of settings. This may partially explain why the model is often used as a guiding philosophy for the care of children, and incorporated with a more structured model, such as Roper, Logan and Tierney's (1996) Activities of Living.

Taking a history from the child and family and conducting a thorough assessment is the start of the process of systematically planning care, which leads to ensuring interventions are appropriate to the individual needs of the child and family. Finally, care must be evaluated, in order to assess the effectiveness of interventions and that it provides opportunity to review the needs of the child and family. Effective documentation is a vital component of care. Documentation of nursing activities is not only a professional requirement (Nursing and Midwifery Council, 2002), but:

- Provides accurate, comprehensive and concise information relating to the child and family
- Provides a record of care required, any problems encountered, interventions and the effectiveness of care

- Provides a baseline upon which the child's condition can be compared

- Is vital in setting and maintaining standards and promoting quality care.

Nash and O'Malley (1997) suggest that comprehensive, concise and easily accessible documentation is essential if there is to be effective communication between departments. This is of particular relevance for the child requiring surgery and is often achieved using a theatre checklist. A checklist may appear to be a task-orientated approach to care. However, information relating to a child's normal routines offers a family-centred approach to care, and recording a child's physiological parameters is not only essential for the safety of the child, but provides opportunity for future comparisons (Heath, 1998). Measuring and documenting the child's physical parameters, in order to ensure that theatre staff have the information necessary to provide optimal care of the child, are vital components of pre-operative care. Height and weight recordings are essential for drug and fluid calculations. Recording the child's baseline temperature, pulse, respirations and blood pressure allow for comparisons both intra and post-operatively. Other parameters, such as baseline oxygen saturations and neurological observations, may be necessary and will depend upon the child's underlying condition and the planned surgical procedure. A typical perioperative care plan, including a theatre check list, is outlined in *Figure 4.1c.*

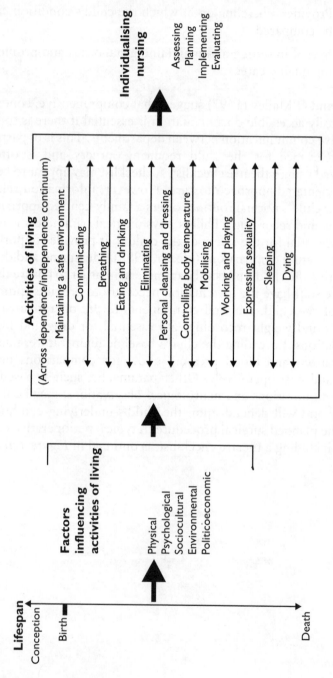

Figure 4.1a: Diagrammatic representation of activities of living model (adapted from Roper, Logan and Tierney, 1996)

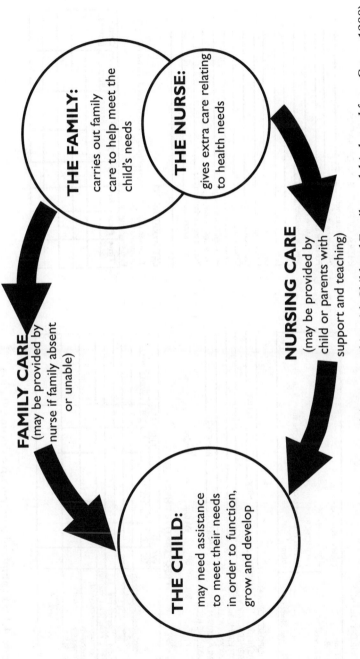

Figure 4.1b: Diagrammatic representation of the Partnership with Child and Family model (adapted from Casey, 1988)

CHILD'S DETAILS

Name	Child's preferred name:
DOB	Child's comforter:
Address	Comforter to remain present in theatre: y/n
	Parents wish to accompany child to the anaesthetic room: y/n
Hospital Number	

PROPOSED OPERATION _____

FASTING: FOOD _____ MILK _____ FLUIDS _____

PREMEDICATION _____

OTHER MEDICATION GIVEN _____

KNOWN ALLERGIES _____

EMLA CREAM: APPLIED _____ REMOVED _____

BASELINE RECORDINGS

T ___ P ___ R ___ BP ___ Weight ___ Height ___ SaO₂ ___

PREOPERATIVE CHECK LIST

	WARD			THEATRE		
	Yes	No	Signature	Yes	No	Signature
Correct identification bands						
Notes						
Prescription chart						
X-Rays (if appropriate)						
Blood results (if appropriate)						
Operation site marked if appropriate						
Presence of loose teeth, cap, brace						
Remove glasses/contact lenses/any prosthesis/jewelry/make-up						

INTRA-OPERATIVE INFORMATION

Type of anaesthetic _____

Positioning during surgery _____

Pressure aids _____

Temperature maintenance _____

Skin preparation _____

Diathermy _____

Laser _____

Drains, catheters, packs _____

Skin closure _____

Ointments/creams _____

Dressings _____

Implants _____

Intra-operative analgesia _____

Local infiltration _____

Procedure performed _____

Special instructions _____

RECOVERY ROOM

To be seen by surgeon/anaesthetist prior to leaving recovery y/n

Intravenous cannula to be left in-situ y/n

Pain relieve prescribed y/n

Time	Pulse	RR	B/P	SaO₂	Pain Score	Sedation Score	Other factors

Figure 4.1c: Example of perioperative documentation

Preparing children physically for theatre and maintaining safety

A major role of the nurse will include the physical preparation of the child for theatre. Care must be timely and appropriate for each individual child and family. Unfortunately, many procedures relating to physical preparation of children for theatre appear to be lacking in evidence or clear rationale. A balance must be achieved between procedures that have safety implications and those that have no apparent value. It is inappropriate to prepare a child for something that is unnecessary, both in terms of the potential distress for the child and family and wasting valuable resources. All aspects of care must be fully explained with appropriate rationale offered, negotiated with the child and family and, where possible, choices given. Many of the traditional practices relating to preparing patients for theatre appear to have their historical roots in attempts to minimise post-operative wound infections (Briggs, 1997). These have commonly included bathing immediately prior to surgery, skin preparation and donning specific theatre clothing. Briggs' review of the literature in relation to reducing skin flora, thus potentially reducing post-operative wound infections, by bath or showering immediately prior to surgery suggests that, unless a skin disinfectant is used, the actual practice has no value. Furthermore, there may be an actual increase in skin flora, thought to be due to a transfer of bacteria from areas of high colonisation, such as the perineum and axilla, to other areas of the body. Briggs (1997) suggests that if the patient desires a bath or shower, then a shower the day prior to surgery is preferable.

Hair removal prior to surgery is not usually an issue in the pre-operative preparation of children. However, it may be relevant for the adolescent requiring surgery. In common with pre-operative bathing, there are no conclusive studies to support the practice of routine hair removal pre-operatively (Briggs, 1997). If hair removal is necessary due to hair becoming entangled with sutures or becoming embedded within the wound itself, with the potential to cause tissue reaction and the formation of a granuloma, then the timing and method of hair removal must be considered. Kjønnisken *et al* (2002), Edlich *et al* (2000),

Briggs (1997) and Small (1996) provide useful reviews of literature relating to hair removal and suggest that when hair removal is necessary, hair clipping or the use of depilatory creams on the day prior to surgery are the method of choice. Shaving with razors causes damage to the skin surface and an increase in transient skin bacteria and should be avoided. The guidelines for hair removal from the Centre for Disease Control and Prevention support these recommendations and advocate that hair removal should only be performed if hair is present at the incision site (Mangram *et al*, 1999). Children may find hair removal procedures unpleasant and it may be more sensitive to undertake these procedures once the child is anaesthetised. Hair removal for cranial surgery is a sensitive issue and needs discussing fully with the child and family in advance of the surgery.

It is difficult to find any literature (relating either to children or adults) concerning the most appropriate choice of clothing for theatre procedures. Presumably traditional theatre gowns have been used because they are clean, easy to remove if necessary, flame resistant and protect the patient's own clothing from the risk of damage due to any spillages that may occur in theatre. Hogg (1994) advocates that children should be permitted to wear their own clothing to theatre and that part of the pre-operative preparation must include providing information relating to the suitability of clothing to bring to hospital (loose, cotton nightwear). If hospital policy dictates or the child and family wish to wear a special gown, these should be designed specifically for children, be available in a range of sizes and protect the privacy and dignity of the child. Children who are distressed should not be coerced against their will to wear a theatre gown. Jewellery is a hazard because of its potential to become caught on theatre equipment and may cause unnecessary injury to the child and theatre personnel. Furthermore, it may act as a conductor and cause skin damage when electrical equipment such as diathermy is used. The need to remove jewellery should be explained to the child and family. If items of jewellery have religious significance, removal must be negotiated with the child and parents; alternatively it may be possible to cover the items with surgical tape in order to minimise the risk of injury. Ideally, all make-up and nail varnish should be removed because of the potential to mask a child's natural colour and react with any substances used in theatre. It is important that any dental bridges or braces are removed, and any loose teeth or capped teeth are recorded and highlighted to the anaesthetist because of the risk of accidental dislodgement and the potential for airway aspiration during intubation.

The child and family must be prepared for medical procedures, and this includes induction of the anaesthesia. The anaesthetist will have discussed and assisted the child and family in the choice of delivery of the anaesthesia, which is usually inhalation induction for infants and young children and intravenous induction for older children and adolescents. Gaining the trust and co-operation of the child and family will greatly assist in ensuring a smooth induction. Unfortunately, as Smalley (1999) highlights, there are still wide variation in practices relating to the preparation of children for medical procedures. This lack of preparation can have long-term consequences for the child; for example, the negative experiences of children undergoing cannulation and venepuncture are contributing to the increase of incidence in needle phobias (Hamilton, 1995). Smalley (1999) suggests that preparation for procedures should include:

- Providing information about the procedure, which should describe the visual, auditory, tactile and olfactory sensations that the child may experience. Honesty is important here, and any potential discomfort should be explained

- Altering aspects of the child's environment, such as involving parents, and a positive, unhurried and supportive attitude of the healthcare professional

- Teaching the child coping strategies, such as using distraction techniques (appropriate to the child's age) and positive reinforcement.

And for cannulation and venepuncture:

- Using topical anaesthetic creams.

Although effective skin analgesia has revolutionised cannulation and venepuncture in children, in order to maximise their potential, it is vital that healthcare professionals choose and apply creams appropriately, and are aware of limitations and complications of topic anaesthetic agents. Emla® (a eutectic mixture of two anesthetic agents: lignocaine and prilocaine), developed in 1980, is probably the most well-known of the topic anaesthetic creams and produces a dermal nerve block if applied to the skin for a minimum of 60 minutes (Fetzer, 2002). Fetzer's meta-analysis of the effectiveness of Emla® suggests that its use has a dramatic effect on the pain experienced during both cannulation and venepuncture in adults and children. Emla® has two main limitations, namely: the recommended application time of 60–90 minutes (Fetzer, 2002; Wolf *et al*, 2002), and not having a license for use in children under one year of age (Meakin and Murat, 2000). The potential complications of Emla® include mild local reactions, such as skin irritation and pallor or erythema, and in the young child, ingestion/aspiration of the occlusive dressing and cream (Norman and Jones, 1990). A secure outer bandage applied over the occlusive dressing is vital for the child at risk of inadvertently displacing the dressing and who is therefore at risk of ingesting the cream (Norman and Jones, 1990). The more severe complication of methaemoglobinaemia, although rare, has a higher potential for developing in children under one year, with the incidence increasing as age decreases (Frayling *et al*, 1990).

An alternative to Emla® is Ametop® (topical amethocaine), which has a shorter action time (30–45 minutes) (Lawson *et al*, 1995) and can be used in children over one month old. Minimal side effects, such as local erythema, have been reported with Ametop® usage (Meakin and Murat, 2000). In view of the benefits of local anaesthesia prior to cannulation and venepuncture, and the relatively lengthy application times of both Emla® and Ametop®, it is understandable that new techniques are being developed. The DPL® (dermal powerject lignocaine) system delivers high velocity lignocaine particles into the skin and has the potential to achieve topical anaesthesia within three minutes (Wolf *et al*, 2002). However, initial results have been inconclusive, particularly with respect to cannulations sited at the back of the hand (Wolf *et al*, 2002). The device is similar in design to a pen injector devise and therefore requires further evaluation in relation to its acceptability in children.

In addition to using appropriate topical analgesia, thoughtful preparation could reduce needle insertion. For example, if bloods are required pre-operatively, rather then performing a venepuncture, a cannula could be inserted and used to administer induction agents.

Traditionally, premedications were administered to improve the safety of anaesthesia (Meakin and Murat, 2000). However, the original rationale for premedications has become less relevant, with improved airway management as anaesthetic techniques have become more sophisticated, the development of new anaesthetic agents and the use of muscle relaxants. The main aims of using a premedication are reducing anxiety and increasing the cooperation of the child (Meakin and Murat, 2000). The frequency of premedication use within the UK has seen a general decline (Mirakhur, 1991) and, with the increase in day surgery, is likely to continue. It is often pre-school children who benefit from sedative premedicants, as this group of children often experiences the greatest stress in an unfamiliar environment and through separation from parents or main carer. The most commonly used premedication in children within the UK is oral trimeprazine (Mirakhur, 1991). Trimeprazine is a long-acting phenothiazine, which has sedative, anticholinergic and anti-emetic properties. However, in some children it can cause increased anxiety, restlessness and distress (Meakin and Murat, 2000). The increasing use of the oral benzodiazepine, midazolam, in the USA (Kain *et al*, 1997), with its short duration of action and reports of less behavioural disturbances (Patel and Meakin, 1997), may result in a change in practice.

Other drugs that may be prescribed pre-operatively include:

- Anticholinergic drugs; for example, atropine, which prevents reflex bradycardia and reduces airway secretion, and may be appropriate for children with excessive secretions or anticipated difficulties in airway management, such as children with cerebral palsy

- H_2 antagonists; for example, cimetidine, which reduces gastric volume and acidity, and may be appropriate in those children at risk of vomiting and regurgitation during anaesthetic induction, such as children with gastro-oesophageal reflux

- Prophylactic antibiotics are indicated for children with cardiac problems, who are at risk of developing bacterial endocarditis

- Pre-emptive analgesics are becoming increasingly popular (McQuay, 1992), and in particular nonsteroidal anti-inflammatory drugs, which are effective if given pre-operatively (Rømsing and Walther-Larsen, 1997).

Fasting prior to surgery

Regurgitation of the stomach contents occurs when the gastric contents flow passively from the stomach into the oesophagus. The normal mechanism of preventing regurgitation, increasing the muscular pressure of the lower oesophagus as the intragastric pressure rises, is rendered ineffective during anaesthesia. Therefore, it is universally accepted that an empty stomach, which safeguards against vomiting, regurgitation and aspiration, is a pre-requisite prior to anaesthesia (Ferrari *et al*, 1999; Sethi *et al*, 1999; Splinter and Schreiner, 1999). Where achievable, the safest method of ensuring the stomach is empty prior to anaesthesia is to have a period of starvation, and is an accepted precondition of elective surgery (Sethi *et al*, 1999). Unfortunately, the effects of pre-operative fasting include hunger, thirst, headache, irritation and discomfort (Sethi *et al*, 1999), which can be traumatic for the child and family. Minimising the length of time children fast has both physiological and psychological benefits (Splinter and Schreiner, 1999). Physiological benefits include: less acidic gastric contents, decreased risk of hypoglycaemia, improved fluid homeostasis and therefore decreased risk of dehydration, decreased lipolysis (Splinter and Schreiner, 1999), and may decrease post-operative nausea and vomiting (Smith *et al*, 1997). Psychologically, the child will be less irritable due to an intake of calories, less thirsty and there will be increased child and parent satisfaction (Splinter and Schreiner, 1999). It is therefore understandable that there has been increased liberalisation of pre-operative fasting times for children in recent years. However, the risk of endangering the safety of the child (primarily the potential for aspiration) must be offset against the need to ensure the child's comfort and preventing complications, such as dehydration and hypoglycaemia (Emerson *et al*, 1998).

The problems in achieving a consensus about the optimal time for fasting children are two-fold; firstly, lack of conclusive evidence in relation to the gastric emptying time for milk, both formula and breast, and solid foods (Ingebo *et al*, 1997; Phillips *et al*, 1994; Splinter and Schreiner, 1999). Secondly, aspiration of stomach contents resulting in pneumonia is thought to occur with stomach volumes above 0.4ml/kg and pH less then 2.5. These volumes have no real scientific basis (Ingebo *et al*, 1997; Phillips *et al*, 1994). Furthermore, they may be less applicable in children, who even after prolonged fasting typically have gastric volumes of greater than 0.4ml/kg and acidic pH levels, and yet have a low occurrence of aspiration during anaesthesia (Ingebo *et al*, 1997; Nicolson and Schreiner, 1994; Phillips *et al*, 1994; Schreiner, 1992). Phillips *et al* undertook a literature review relating to the incidence and pathogenesis of regurgitation in children, the relationship of gastro-oesohageal reflux and aspiration pneumonitis, the relationship between fasting and the risk of aspiration and discusses the advantages of short fasting times. There does not appear to be conclusive evidence to support the length of the traditional fast time of six hours for clear fluids. The studies reviewed by Phillips *et al* and, more recently, Splinter and Schreiner (1999) indicate that a two-hour fast time in children for clear fluids is sufficient to ensure an acceptable pH and residual gastric volume for the safe induction of anaesthesia.

Although there is evidence to support a fast of two hours for clear fluids, with clear fluids being defined as water, fruit juices which do not contain pulp, clear tea or coffee (American Society of Anesthetists, 1999), there are no conclusive studies in relation to the optimal fast time for breast milk, formula and solid food (Ingebo *et al*, 1997; Phillips *et al*, 1994; Nicolson and

Schreiner, 1994; Schreiner, 1992; Splinter and Schreiner, 1999). This is of particular importance in the child health setting, because of the practicalities of caring for children. For example, the majority of neonates and young infants, who take a milk feed 3–4 hourly, refuse and are not satisfied by clear fluids (Sethi, 1999). These children will be at risk of hypoglycaemia if fasted for the traditional six hours. Early studies by Cavell (1979) indicated that the emptying half-life of breast milk from the stomach is 25 minutes, and that of formula milk 50 minutes. However, Sethi *et al*'s (1999) more recent preliminary study, using real-time ultrasound, assessed the gastric emptying time of glucose, low fat formula, and breast milk in children under five years of age. Their results suggest that glucose and formula can be given safely to children at two hours and three hours respectively, but that breast milk had a slower emptying time than formula. The results were statistically inconclusive, and contradict more traditional views; therefore, and understandably, the researchers would not recommend a fasting time for breast milk. Furthermore, caution needs to be applied when making generalisations from available studies; for example, infant formula can vary greatly in composition with wide variations in relation to fat content (Splinter and Schreiner, 1999).

There appears to be the least amount of evidence available investigating the ingestion of solid food and its relationship to pre-operative fasting in children (American Society of Anesthetists, 1999; Phillips *et al*, 1994; Splinter and Schreiner, 1999). Furthermore, as Phillips *et al* highlight, there is no absolute definition of a solid, citing the examples of gelatin, which is a solid but promptly liquefies on entering the stomach, and milk, which is a liquid but separates into whey (remaining liquid) and curds (a solid) in the stomach. The need to treat milk as a solid has implications in the child health setting. The emptying time of food from the stomach will undoubtedly be influenced by the composition of the food ingested, and depend upon the proportions of fats, carbohydrates and proteins. The American Society of Anesthetists Task Force (American Society of Anesthetists, 1999) defines a light meal as toast (or similar foodstuff) and a drink, with a recommended fast time of six hours, and a complex meal as one that contains fried or fatty foods. Complex meals can take over eight hours to leave the stomach, and therefore a recommended fast of a minimum of eight hours is advocated.

Recent guidelines by the Association of Anaesthetists (2001) within the UK recommend the following fasting guidelines for children undergoing elective surgery:

- *Neonates and infants*: two hours clear fluids; four hours breast milk; six hours formula milk and solids
- *Children*: two hours clear fluids; six hours formula milk and solids.

The times recommended are not supported by conclusive research, but represent a combination of evaluating the evidence available and peer consensus. Fasting guidelines require monitoring through the audit cycle in terms of adherence to the guidelines and occurrence of aspiration, because the presence of guidelines alone are not enough to change practice (Emerson *et al*, 1998).

Bates (1994) undertook an audit of fasting within a children's day care setting following the introduction of guidelines recommending a two-hour fluid fast. The results highlighted wide variation in the fasting times of children, and of particularly concern were the 31 percent of the children who had fasted for 12 hours or more. Factors which contributed to the length of the fast included blanket written instructions; for example, instructions based on adult practices (12 midnight fast for the morning list and to fast following a light breakfast for the afternoon list), incorrect information being sent to parents, and all children fasting for the same length of time regardless of their position on the theatre list. Changes in practice, such as more specific and individualised written instructions and assessing whether the child was able to have a drink immediately on arrival on the unit, dramatically reduced these excessive fast times. A repeat audit demonstrated the maximum time any child fasted was 4.5 hours, compared to 17 hours in the first audit.

Although adherence to fasting guidelines is a way forward to ensure children are not excessively fasted, it is imperative that each child is assessed as an individual. Phillips *et al*'s (1994) review of the literature suggests than the incidence of perioperative pulmonary aspiration is rare (0.001–0.009%) and more likely to be associated with:

- Emergency surgery
- Surgery performed out of normal working hours
- Presence of factors which delay stomach emptying, such as obesity, raised intra-cranial pressure, gastrointestinal disease, stress, pain, trauma
- Conditions where there is increased risk of regurgitation, such as gastro-oesophageal reflux, renal failure and diabetes
- Impaired bronchial clearing, such as altered consciousness, bulbar palsy
- Inexperienced anaesthetist.

In addition, certain medication may have an effect upon gastric emptying, and is relevant to both premedications and the child's regular medication (Splinter and Schreiner, 1999). For example, opioids and anticholinergic drugs are thought to delay stomach emptying, while trimeprazine appears to reduce gastric contents, and midazolam does not appear to have any effect on gastric contents. It is generally accepted that the majority of children should continue to take their regular medication as normal prior to surgery. Any doubts should be discussed with the appropriate anaesthetist. For children at risk of regurgitation, the anaesthetist should consider procedures that minimise potential complications (American Society of Anesthetists, 1999; Phillips *et al*, 1994), such as increasing the length of the fasting period, gastric aspiration via a naso-gastric tube, using H_2 antagonists (e.g. cimetidine), using antacids (e.g. sodium citrate), rapid sequence induction and tracheal intubation, as appropriate to the clinical situation. Ensuring that a child is assessed as an individual and fasted appropriately is a vital component of pre-operative care. If the child and family are to receive appropriate and consistent support and care, and be involved in the decision-making process, the multidisciplinary team must understand the general principles of pre-operative fasting and apply these to the individual child. If the care between departments is to be seamless, then it is imperative that healthcare professionals communicate effectively and any child at risk of being inappropriately fasted highlighted quickly to ensure prompt and appropriate action is taken.

Transport to theatre

In order to ensure seamless care, maintain safety and encourage parental involvement, it is essential that cohesive protocols exist for transporting children to theatre, and that there is effective inter-departmental communication. Some theatre suites have a holding bay to reduce delays between cases. It is essential these areas consider the psychological well-being of the child and that facilities are appropriate; for example, a child-friendly environment with a range of play facilities/activities to meet all ages, the area to be separate from adult waiting areas and that parents are made to feel welcome and included. In addition, the waiting time for children following arrival in the theatre suite and induction of the anaesthetic should be kept to a minimum (Hogg, 1994).

It is essential that the journey to theatre does not contribute to the child's anxiety (Hogg, 1994). Therefore it is vital that the child is offered appropriate choices, which should be appropriate to his/her age and condition. Children who have had a sedative premedication will require to be escorted on a theatre trolley or on their own bed. Theatre trolleys can be made interesting for the young child, for example by depicting modes of transport from popular children's characters, such as Thomas the Tank Engine. It has become increasingly common for children who have not had a sedative premedication to walk to theatre or, if an infant, to be carried by their parent. The use of motorised toy cars can be an exciting prospect for the pre-school child. Parents should be given the choice of accompanying their child to theatre, and the child should be encouraged to take his/her favourite toy, book or comforter with him or her.

4.2   Intra-operative care

It is usual practice prior to leaving the ward to ensure the correct child is being escorted to theatre for the correct operation, that all pre-operative requirements have been met, and the identification of the child is confirmed (*Figure 4.1c*). This information should be confirmed again prior to induction of the anaesthesia (Walker and Lockie, 2000). In addition, this is an opportunity for ward staff to highlight information relating to each individual child, such as any known allergies, pain relief already administered, and specific details relating to the child and family, which may be of value to the theatre staff in the intra-operative phase. The actual intra-operative phase begins when the child arrives in the anaesthetic room.

The anaesthetic room

Hogg's (1994: 21) standard for children undergoing surgery in relation to the anaesthetic room states that, 'the environment and procedures in the anaesthetic room should minimise the anxiety of the child and family'. In order to achieve this standard, the environment should not appear threatening; therefore sights, smells and sounds that may be distressing to the child should be minimised. The decor should be child-friendly, unnecessary medical equipment should not be visible, and there should be a range of appropriate and suitable play/distraction activities. Furthermore, a parent should be encouraged, but not pressurised, to remain with the child (Hogg, 1994). This requires the area having enough space to accommodate the parent and a ward nurse, while maintaining a safe environment in which theatre staff can work effectively. Unfortunately, there are wide discrepancies relating to supporting parents' wishes to be present during the induction of anaesthesia (Meakin and Murat, 2000).

The practice appears to be more acceptable within the UK (McCormick and Spargo, 1996) and perhaps reflects Department of Health (1991) recommendations that the presence of parents during all aspects of care, and in particular where situations may be stressful (for example, investigation and induction of anaesthesia), should not be viewed as a luxury. Allowing parents in the anaesthetic room avoids the distress that separation from parents can bring and has the potential to reduce both the child's immediate anxiety and long-term behaviour problems. Unfortunately, there is only limited evidence to support these claims, which is often based on 'best practice' rather than rigorous research (Glasper and Powell, 2000). The reasons for excluding parents from the anaesthetic room have been cited as the greater potential for a difficult induction in children, particularly children under one year of age or children with serious pre-existing disease, and children presenting as an emergency (Hannallah and Epstein, 1991). Advocates of parental inclusion may find these barriers tenuous and therefore inappropriate. Attempts to determine the benefits in terms of reducing a child's anxiety on induction of anaesthetic have, in general, been inconclusive and, perhaps unsurprisingly, showed variations across the age span (Kain et al, 2000; 1996). Parents included in the anaesthetic room indicate a greater satisfaction with the separation process and the overall quality of the service offered (Kain et al, 2000). Children who do not respond well to new situations may react better to having a parent present. The presence of a parent in the anaesthetic room does not appear to increase the length of the induction nor the safety of the procedure (Kain et al, 1996). The decision to include a parent must consider the child's and parents' wishes in conjunction with discussions with the anaesthetist.

The role of the nurse in the theatre environment is changing to include specialist practice, such as the surgeon's assistant, where some surgical interventions are undertaken, and the anaesthetist's assistant, where anaesthetic assessment, airway management and discharge from recovery are undertaken (Boss, 2002; Cowan, 1998; Wise, 1999). The core role of the nurse in the theatre environment is to ensure the anaesthetic, surgical and recovery needs of the patient are met (Cowan, 1998; Wise, 1999). This is achieved by co-ordinating the activities of the multidisciplinary team, supervising the whole experience of the patient, and assessing, planning, implementing and evaluating care (Cowan, 1998; Wise, 1999). This requires knowledge and skills relating to anaesthetic and surgical techniques, post-anaesthetic care, infection control management, maintaining a safe environment, risk assessment and pain management. In the paediatric setting, the role will include being an advocate for the child and family, ensuring guidelines are appropriate to meet the needs of the child and are audited, being competent with equipment specifically designed for children, and keeping up-to-date with current child care issues and practices.

Principles of anaesthesia

The purpose of anaesthesia is to ensure that the surgery can proceed under the optimal conditions and to keep the child comfortable. However, anaesthesia is not without risks, with deaths in children largely confined to high-risk groups, where children have complex and multiple problems, or adverse drug reactions (National Confidential Enquiry into Perioperative Deaths, 1999). Anaesthesia in children has particular challenges due to physiological, anatomical and psychological differences from adults, with the most significant differences occurring in the neonatal period. Modern anaesthesia is composed of the triad of inducing unconsciousness, achieving effective muscle relaxation, and the provision of suitable analgesia. The drugs and techniques used affect all vital body systems, with loss of all modalities of sensation, such as pain, touch, temperature and position, and in the case of general anaesthesia, there is an associated loss of consciousness. Children have a low residual respiratory capacity, a high minute ventilation and cardiac output, a high metabolic rate and a large body surface area in relation to weight; therefore patho-physiological changes, such as hypoxia, hypercarbia, hypovolaemia and hypothermia, can occur quickly. Paediatric anaesthesia has developed as a specialty within its own right. Within the UK, the principles of ensuring a quality anaesthetic service is provided to all children have been clearly identified by the Royal College of Anaesthetists (2001) and include:

- Care must be delivered by appropriately trained medical and nursing staff

- Special facilities for certain groups of children, such as neonates (less than 44 weeks gestation), children with significant co-morbidity and children with complex surgical needs, including major trauma

- A consultant who regularly anaesthetises children should lead the service

- There must be a child-centred approach to care, which includes facilities separate from adult patients, parental involvement in all aspects of care, appropriate consent and consideration of the rights of the child

- The availability of appropriate paediatric equipment

- A properly funded and staffed acute pain service specifically for children

- Occasional paediatric practice is unacceptable.

Although most of the responsibility for anaesthetic services has been designated to the paediatric anaesthetist, it is essential that all professionals caring for children in the perioperative period have a general understanding of the principles behind anaesthetic techniques and the effects of drug combinations used.

Inhalation or intravenous are the most common methods of inducing anaesthesia in children (Walker and Lockie, 2000). Inhalation anaesthesia is achieved by providing a combination of oxygen and vaporised anaesthetic gases. These gases travel from the lungs to the brain and result in unconsciousness. Typically, nitrous oxide is used as an adjunct to a volatile anaesthetic agent, such as Sevoflurane® or Halothane®, for induction purposes. Maintaining on Sevoflurane® or Halothane® or changing to Isoflurane® or desflurane then achieves ongoing anaesthesia. Although there are variations in practice, it has been suggested that Isoflurane® and desflurane have a low metabolism (Eger, 1994) and are more cost effective (Walker and Lockie, 2000). However, they are less suitable for induction because of their pungent smell and the need to increase concentration slowly, which can result in increased irritability in the child's airway (Walker and Lockie, 2000). Masks impregnated with different flavours and play devised to encourage children to tolerate face-masks are valuable in gaining the child's co-operation.

Although the number of anaesthetic agents is ever increasing, the two most commonly used intravenous anaesthetic agents in children are probably thiopentone and proprofol (Booker, 2000; Walker and Lockie, 2000). Both have a rapid onset time, but thiopentone has a longer recovery time than proprofol, making it less suitable for surgery of a short duration. Propofol's main disadvantages are pain on injection and not having a licence for use in children under three years of age. It does, however, have a relatively low incidence of nausea and vomiting (Walker and Lockie, 2000). Walker and Lockie provide a useful review of the advantages and disadvantages of inhalation versus intravenous induction of anaesthesia (*Table 4.2a*).

Table 4.2a: Advantages and disadvantages of inhalation versus intravenous induction of anaesthesia (adapted from Walker and Lockie, 2000)

Factor	Inhalation induction	Intravenous induction
Hypoxia	Pre-oxygenation can reduce hypoxia. Irritation of anaesthetic gases may result in coughing or laryngospasm making intubation difficult. Needs experienced staff, one to manage the airway once child is anaesthetised and one to obtain venous access.	Possible increased risk of hypoxia than with inhalation techniques, particularly in the child with a difficult or partially obstructed airway.
Over-dosage	Can occur if effects of gases are not effectively monitored or not reduced once anaesthesia has been achieved, with resultant depression of cardiovascular and respiratory systems.	Can occur due to miscalculation of dosages, with resultant depression of cardiovascular and respiratory systems.
Psychological effects	Children may have vivid memories of the procedure, which may have implications if further surgery is required.	Often well accepted if topical anaesthetic creams are used. Often long-term effects will depend upon the smoothness of the cannulation. Not suitable in children with needle phobias.
Overall acceptability	Failure is less common than with intravenous induction. Child must remain fairly motionless either on parent's lap or on a trolley and accept having a face mask or either held close or over their face. Needs effective communication and swift transition for transferring a child from parent's lap to the trolley.	Needs to have secure venous access to be successful. Limb in which venous access is to be established needs to be held firm, which may be more acceptable than holding for inhalation induction.Drugs may cause pain on injection.

If there is no strong clinical evidence for either method, the child and family may choose and some children may have strong preferences. Children are more vulnerable to upper airway obstruction than adults. The need to maintain a patent airway is a vital part of the care of the child both intra- and post-operatively. Maintaining the airway during surgery is the primary concern of the anaesthetist. Because of the potential for airway problems in children, and the need for recovery staff to be competent in maintaining the airway for all age ranges in childhood, all staff caring for the anaesthetised child and the child recovering from anaesthesia require the knowledge and skills to manage potential airway problems. Furthermore, in order to support the anaesthetist, familiarity with techniques is vital in ensuring the smooth management of the child in the theatre environment. The choice of airway management in the anaesthetised child will depend upon the age of the child, the surgical procedure, ventilation requirements and the presence of any pre-existing airway/respiratory problems. The main types of airway management include facemask (with or without an airway), laryngeal mask and endotracheal intubation (Walker and Lockie, 2000). Basic airway management is discussed in *Chapter 3*.

The use of muscle relaxants has greatly benefited many surgical procedures by ensuring a motionless environment in which the surgeons work, and is usually a requirement prior to endotracheal intubation (Walker and Lockie, 2000). Many surgical procedures in children are of a fairly short duration, for example herniotomies, orchidopexies and tonsillectomies, and, depending upon the surgical techniques used, may not require the use of a muscle relaxants. Muscle relaxants prevent movement, but they do not have analgesic properties nor have any effects upon conscious levels. The range of muscle relaxants now available has allowed the anaesthetist to accurately predict the duration of their action (Goudsouzian, 2000). Succinycholine is probably the most widely used short-acting, depolarising muscle relaxant (Goudsouzian, 2000) and, despite side-effects, including bradyarryhmias, hyperkalaemia, masseter spasm and, more rarely, reports of increased incidence of myoglobinuria, malignant hyperthermia and cardiac arrest, is often used to assist in tracheal intubation. Intermediate action muscle relaxants include atricurium, cisatracurium, and vecuronium, and are often given as a single dose on induction and topped up as necessary. There are relatively few side-effects (Goudsouzian, 2000). However, non-depolarising relaxants require their action reversing to coincide with the end of the surgical procedure using a neuromuscular antagonist such as neostigmine. Pancuronium has been a popular long-acting muscle relaxant in children (Goudsouzian, 2000) because of the tendency to cause a slight tachycardia and hence ensure a good cardiac output. Other long-acting muscle relaxants include pipecuronium and doxacurium. Again, these non-depolarising muscle relaxants require their action reversing at the end of the procedure. The clinical signs of recovery from all muscle relaxants must be monitored and include satisfactory respiratory effort, facial movements, limb movements and vocal sounds, such as crying.

Effective pain management is an essential component of the care of the child undergoing surgery. Although effective pain management is dependent upon a multidisciplinary approach, in practice, the overall responsibility of post-operative pain management is devolved, certainly in terms of immediate post-operative planning and prescribing analgesia regimes, to the paediatric anaesthetist (Howard and Lloyd-Thomas, 2000). Pain management is discussed in *Chapter 5*; it is worth outlining the contribution local anaesthesia makes to post-operative pain management. Local anaesthetic agents, such as bupivacaine and ropivacaine, injected around a nerve or group of nerves will block the pain impulses to the region of the body those nerves supply. Commonly performed nerve blocks in children, include:

- Inguinal block, which is suitable for inguinal hernia repairs and orchidopexies

- Penile block, which is suitable for circumcision

- Axillary block, which is suitable for arm and hand surgery

- Femoral block, which is suitable for surgery to femur and thigh

- Caudal block, which is suitable for surgery below umbilicus.

It is usual practice to inject local anaesthetics at the beginning of a procedure, with the usual duration of effectiveness being 4–6 hours. If oral analgesics are given when the child is able to tolerate them and to coincide with the reduction in the effectiveness of the local block, successful levels of analgesia can be achieved. The advantages of local anaesthetic nerve blocks include the ability to achieve effective analgesia without systemic drug effects and they do not potentiate the effects of general anaesthetics drugs. Children and their families should be warned of the potential for leg weakness following caudal, femoral and inguinal nerve blocks.

It is of vital importance that staff have knowledge of pain assessment and management in children. Post-operative pain assessment should begin as soon as the child arrives in recovery, in order to ensure that the child receives prompt and appropriate care. The presence of pain will complicate recovery. Leaving pain management until the child reaches the ward is not acting in the best interests of the child (Department of Health, 1989) and, as pain intensity increases, the management becomes much more difficult. Recovery staff must ensure assessment and interventions are documented and that pain management plans are clearly documented and articulated to the nurse taking over the care of the child following discharge from recovery.

Maintaining a safe environment

The safety of the child, minimising risks and the early detection of complications are essential components of care within the theatre environment and include:

- Ensuring the correct positioning of the child
- Implementing interventions to prevent injury and relieve pressure during procedures
- Implementing infection control measures
- Minimising heat loss and maintaining body temperature
- Identification of potential problems
- Effective observation and monitoring of the child.

An important role for theatre staff includes ensuring procedures relating to infection control are instigated and maintained, because the major source of post-operative wound contamination appears to occur during the actual surgical procedure (Horwitz *et al*, 1998). Practices that help to minimise wound contamination, include (Gould, 2001):

- Ensuring the environment is cleaned thoroughly, including all surfaces, walls and floors

- Dealing with spillages promptly and appropriately

- Maintaining ventilation systems in compliance with manufacturers' recommendations

- Adhering to policies and procedures related to clothing, wearing of masks, gowns and use of gloves, and guidelines for managing infections

- Maintaining strict asepsis and equipment sterility during operations

- Minimising the movement and number of personnel within theatres

- Ensuring adequate skin preparation.

During surgery, observations of the child's physiological status will, as a minimum, include: monitoring the heart rate and rhythms, blood pressure, respiratory rate and effort, skin colour, oxygen saturation levels, consciousness levels and temperature. A range of equipment will be utilised for monitoring the child's physical condition, which should supplement clinical observations and allow for the prompt detection of changes. It is essential that equipment maintenance adheres to safety legislation, and that all staff are competent in the use of the equipment within their area. Due to the stresses placed upon the physiological systems of the child in the theatre environment, effective monitoring and prompt interventions are vital. Further, compromises may occur from drug reactions and, more recently, the increasing development of latex allergies (Burns, 1997), both of which may cause anaphylaxis.

Infants and children do not have the same ability as adults to maintain body temperature (Noble *et al*, 1997) due to the higher ratio of surface area to body weight, less subcutaneous fat, and thinner dermis and epidermis. Intra-operatively, the ability to maintain a normal body temperature is compromised (Imrie and Hall, 1990), because:

- General anaesthetic agents impair normal thermoregulatory responses, probably due to attenuation of hypothalamic function

- There is a reduction in the metabolic rate

- Of increased thermal losses due to skin exposure, which can be significant in the young child

- Of low ambient temperatures

- Of administration of cold intravenous fluids, drugs and skin preparation fluids

- Of risk of developing malignant hyperthermia, which can be triggered by some anaesthetic agents.

Children who become hypothermic are at a greater risk of hypoxaemia and hypercapnoea, and have a more prolonged recovery period (Olsson, 2000). Measures that should be instigated to reduce heat loss include: ensuring the child is adequately insulated with blankets, use of warming mattresses, use of radiant heaters, minimal exposure of skin surfaces, anaesthetic gases and fluids are warmed, the ambient temperature is appropriate, and the child's temperature is regularly monitored (Imrie and Hall, 1990). In an ideal situation and to estimate total body temperature, both core and peripheral temperatures would need to be recorded. In practice, this rarely occurs (Imrie and Hall, 1990). Oesophageal, rectal, tympanic membrane and axilla skin probes are commonly used to estimate body temperature (Noble *et al*, 1997).

Malignant hyperthermia is an inherited disorder of skeletal muscle, in which the muscles increase their metabolic rate, oxygen consumption and production of lactate acid (Noble *et al*, 1997), and can be triggered by some anaesthetic agents.

Although the pathophysiology is not clearly understood, the symptoms include: increased temperature, tachycardia, tachypnoea, arrhythmias, cyanosis, muscle rigidity and labile blood pressure, and can lead to a hypermetabolic crisis (Pritchard, 2003). Although a rare condition with an estimated incidence of 1 in 15 000 children (Pritchard, 2003), due to its potentially fatal nature, early detection and prompt treatment of the condition are essential. Children at risk of developing malignant hyperthermia, such as those with a first-degree relative diagnosed as having malignant hyperthermia, must be referred to a recognised centre and undergo investigations to determine if they have the disorder. Diagnosis is primarily by identification of contractures in muscle tissue obtained by biopsy, then exposure to halothane or caffeine (Pritchard, 2003). Once diagnosed, the child must always receive anaesthetic and muscle relaxant drugs that do not trigger a crisis, such as nitrous oxide and pancuronium. If a crisis occurs, early management includes:

- Withdrawing anaesthetic drugs and installing a clean re-breath system

- Abandoning surgery if possible

- Administration of dantrolene (reduces muscle tone and metabolic rate)

- Hyperventilation with oxygen

- Using cooling measures to manage temperature

- Measuring arterial blood gases, potassium and creatine phosphokinase

- Close cardiovascular and temperature monitoring.

(Pritchard, 2003)

Once the initial crisis has been managed, the child will probably require intensive management to monitor and treat potential problems, such as arrhythmias, hyperkalaemia, or metabolic acidosis. The child and family will require ongoing counselling, support and advice in relation to future anaesthetics.

Recovery from anaesthesia

The aim of care in the immediate post-operative period is to prevent potential life-threatening complications following anaesthesia and surgery (Heath, 1998). Post-operative complications may occur at any stage, but are more likely to occur in the immediate stage of recovery and include airway obstruction, hypoxaemia, bleeding, agitation/delirium, hypothermia, and nausea and vomiting (Watcha, 2000). It is essential that staff caring for children in this early stage have excellent observation and assessment skills, and that staffing levels reflect the dependency level of the child. Therefore, the immediate post-operative care usually takes place in a designated recovery area within the theatre suite. Although most children will be breathing spontaneously on arrival in the recovery area, the residual effects of drugs administered during anaesthesia may still be present, and the child may not have complete control of the airway and might be at risk of airway obstruction. Until the gag and cough reflex return to normal, the child will be unable to clear his/her airway and pooling of secretions may further compromise the airway. Opioids and neuromuscular blocking agents can cause respiratory depression. Children will require airway management and a high degree of monitoring until safely recovered from anaesthesia, and this should include observations of conscious levels, respiratory rate and effort, oxygen saturation levels, and cardiovascular monitoring (skin colour, skin temperature, pulse and blood pressure) and temperature. The frequency of observations will depend upon the initial assessment of the child, duration and type of surgery, and drugs used. An essential element of care in the immediate post-operative period is the early detection of shock and haemorrhage by observing for changes in colour, pulse and blood pressure, and immediate blood loss from the wound site/dressings. The management of shock and haemorrhage is described in *Chapter 3*.

Relatively new is the practice of supporting parents, if they so wish, to be present in the recovery area as soon as practicably possible; the success of these practices appears beneficial (Brown, 1997; 1995; Fina *et al*; 1997). Benefits include: reduced anxiety in the child, early involvement of the parents in the post-operative care of their child, particularly in providing comfort and reassurance, facilitating an altogether less traumatic experience for the child and family (Brown, 1995). The major obstacle appears to be concerns about the provision of information to the parents, if the procedure has not gone according to plan (Brown, 1995). One of the first questions a parent will undoubtedly ask is, if the procedure went without complications. This will occur regardless of whether parents are first reunited with their child on the ward or in the recovery area. It is usual practice for the surgeon who has carried out the procedure to explain to parents the nature and potential outcome of any complications. It is essential this communication takes place as soon as possible and, in practical terms, is often much easier to facilitate in the recovery area, where the surgeon can be on hand prior to the next case starting, with only minimal disruption to the theatre list (Brown, 1995). To ensure their presence is maximised, parents should have clear expectations of their role within recovery and an understanding of what to expect. Other considerations within the recovery area include: ensuring there is adequate space to accommodate parents to ensure that safety of the child is not compromised, equipment and decor should be appropriate for a child, and children should have a recovery area separated from adult patients (Hogg, 1994).

As soon as practically possible, the child should be returned to the familiar ward environment. Children should only be discharged from recovery when able to maintain their own airway, they have regained a satisfactory level of consciousness, and all physiological parameters are stable. The handover to the ward staff must be of sufficient depth to ensure that communications (both written and verbal) relating to the specific condition and post-operative needs, including pain management plans, are clearly articulated to the member of staff accepting the responsibility of the child. There should be a policy for the transfer of the child from the recovery room to the ward, including type of equipment available on the transporting trolley, i.e. as a minimum, oxygen and suction, and the level and experience of escorting staff, who must be capable of dealing with any emergency situation that might arise during transfer.

4.3 Post-operative care

Preparation for receiving a child back from theatre on to the ward begins prior to the child's arrival, with preparation of the bed space and necessary monitoring equipment. As a minimum, this should include ease of access from the theatre trolley to the bed, and ensuring oxygen and suction are readily available and in working order. Specific equipment should be anticipated for planned procedures and prepared, for example infusion stands, advanced monitoring equipment, drain and catheter holders, and relevant documentation. There needs to be consideration of the child's on position the ward, which must be appropriate for the child's needs and for the predicted level of observation required.

Physical safety

Ensuring the child's physical safety will be the first priority on return to the ward. The initial assessment of the post-operative patient usually consists of recording vital signs (respiration, pulse, blood pressure and temperature) and general assessment relating to consciousness levels, ability to maintain an airway, colour, presence of swallow reflex, discharge and appearance of dressings/wound, pain levels, and presence of nausea, and specific consideration relating to the type of surgery, such as intravenous infusions, catheters and drains (Zeitz and McCutcheon, 2002).

The purpose of undertaking post-operative observations is to detect complications (Zeitz and McCutcheon, 2002) and, in the case of recording vital signs, ensuring that physiological functions, altered during anaesthesia, are returning to normal limits. Although the potential for adverse events relating to anaesthesia will decrease with time, it cannot be assumed that discharge from recovery occurs when the child is completely free from potential risk of airway obstruction, shock and haemorrhage. However, the potential problems that may occur in this stage of recovery are more likely to include haemorrhage, nausea and vomiting, pain, dizziness and excessive drowsiness (Watcha, 2000). The frequency of observations in the ward environment will depend upon many factors, such as type of surgery, length of surgery, responsiveness of the child upon return to the ward, presence of advanced analgesia systems (such as opioid infusions) and the initial assessment.

Zeitz and McCutcheon's (2002) review of policies and procedures relating to undertaking vital signs post-operatively showed great diversity, in terms of both the type and frequency of the observations. Nurses base their practice on what they **believe** is hospital policy (Botti and Hunt, 1994) and traditional task-orientated models of care (Burroughs and Hoffbrand, 1990), rather than linked to individual patient need. While policies do appear to exist in relation to the frequency of recording vital signs post-operatively, statements are vague, lacking sufficient information to guide practice and too generalised for use in many clinical situations (Zeitz and McCutcheon, 2002). It would appear that policies relating to recording of vital signs following routine surgical procedures relate to the first 24 hours post theatre, with the most common regime being to record a minimum of pulse and respirations one-hourly for four hours, then reduced to four hourly. The recording of pulse and respirations appears to be deemed an essential component of vital signs, whereas blood pressure and temperature-taking are secondary considerations and therefore performed less frequently—i.e. four hourly. There is no indication whether the policies reviewed by Zeitz and McCutcheon (2002) were age-specific. However, there appears to be a dearth of published data relating to the frequency of observations in children. The most important consideration is to ensure the type and frequency of observations meet the needs of the child and that nurses can identify clear rationales for their decision-making processes. Although this may be difficult in the absence of current evidence, nurses need to consider the potential risk of the likelihood of complications occurring; the safety of the child balanced with performing unnecessary procedures and causing undue distress. In addition, nurses will need to adapt practice in relation to the age and stage of development of the child, an example being the increased risk of apnoea and bradycardia, due to immature physiological responses in the neonatal period (Steward, 1982; Welborn et al, 1986). It would seem logical that these infants will require more frequent observations and continuous monitoring to detect apnoeic episodes and episodes of bradycardia.

Post-operative nausea and vomiting (PONV) is a major issue post anaesthesia, because of the distress it causes and the incidence (estimated at between 40–50 percent), and is one of the most frequently cited reasons for delayed discharge from hospital (Cohen *et al*, 1990; Lerman, 1992). If severe, PONV can put additional strain on the wound and contribute to bleeding. PONV is more likely:

- To occur in children than in adults
- Where there have been high levels of preoperative anxiety, in association with certain surgical procedures (such as ophthalmic surgery, inner ear surgery, dental surgery, abdominal surgery)
- When opioids have been used
- When there has been insufflation of the stomach during anaesthesia.

(Burns, 1997)

In addition, the introduction of fluids early in the post-operative period and early mobilisation may contribute to PONV. Kearney *et al* (1998) undertook a randomised control trial in order to investigate PONV in children. The control group ingested oral fluids post-operatively as soon as the child chose to drink (in the majority of cases around 60 minutes post-operatively), with the study group encouraged to withhold from taking fluids until after 4–6 hours post-operatively. The results showed PONV occurred in 56 percent of children in the control group and 38 percent in the study group. Although the results were statistically significant, there are some limitations to the study; for example, children admitted for day care were discharged without the need to have taken fluids, if they met all other discharge criteria, and may have vomited at home. Furthermore, adopting the practice of withholding fluids has implications for practice, such as increasing the responsibility of parents if discharge occurs prior to the requirement of tolerating oral fluids. Discharge criteria would require modification for day surgery and there would need to be a compensatory volume of intravenous fluids given during theatre in order to minimise the risk of dehydration. Patients' compliance in Kearney *et al*'s (1998) study was excellent, but there would need to be greater exploration of the potential to cause distress if children have fluids withheld for a significant length of time post-operatively.

Watcha (2000) suggests that minimising PONV is a vital component of care for the child undergoing anaesthesia. In light of limited evidence to support clear guidance in relation to the timing and type of fluid/foods to be offered to a child post-operatively, common sense needs to prevail. PONV can be reduced by:

- Avoidance of premedications and anaesthetic agents that are known to increase the risk of PONV

- Consideration of alternative pain management to opioids, which are known to increase PONV, particularly for day surgery and minor procedures, such as local anaesthetic and nerve blocks, and non-steroidal anti-inflammatory drugs

- Administering anti-emetic drugs prophylactically intra-operatively for procedures where there is a high risk of PONV

- Providing sufficient fluid intra-operatively

- Not rushing a child to drink post-operatively, while not withholding fluids from a distressed child (unless surgery indicates the child must remain nil by mouth)

- Preventing large volumes of fluids being ingested over a short span of time and, where possible, avoiding fluids with increased acidity, such as fruit juices/fizzy drinks.

Nausea and vomiting can be distressing for the child and family, and if severe can lead to dehydration. The child and family will require support and reassurance. Treatment with anti-emetic drugs may be necessary.

Other surgical complications will relate to the type of surgery; for example, splints and dressings may be tight in orthopaedic problems, resulting in compartment syndromes developing, and urinary problems and catheter blockages can develop following urological procedures.

Psychological care

Continuing support and collaborative working with the child are essential elements of post-operative care. The principles of ensuring effective communication, described pre-operatively, will continue to apply, and although the child and family should have been prepared for post-operative procedures, these will need re-explaining. Preparation for post-operative procedures, appropriate to the child's age and stage of development, is just as important in the post- as pre-operative period. This is particularly important if the child has to undergo repeated procedures, such as regular venepuncture or dressing changes. Equipment that will be required post-operatively should have been explained and where possible shown to the child and family in advance. This will need re-visiting as soon as practically possible after theatre. Continued parental involvement and, where possible, giving choices are vital in ensuring the child feels he/she has some degree of independence and control of treatments and care.

Ongoing care and preparation for discharge

Children and parents need to be prepared for the care required after surgery (Hogg, 1994). There appears to be a lack of consensus relating to many aspects of general care following surgery, such as when the child can mobilise, eat and drink, bath and return to school. However, all these elements will apply to most children and will be issues that the child and family will require information about.

Nursing staff should not coerce a child into drinking early post-operative, but encourage small volumes of non-acidic fluid when the child starts to become thirsty. Food can be introduced once oral fluids have been tolerated. Unless the type of surgery restricts mobility, then the child should be allowed to rest and not rushed into early mobilisation. If a caudal, femoral or inguinal nerve block has been used, it is important to check that there is no weakness in the legs prior to mobilisation. Briggs' (1997) review of the literature suggests that once the wound edges are sealed (usually within 48 hours) then bathing will not affect wound healing or increase the likelihood of a wound infection developing. However, a shower may be preferable to a bath because there will be less susceptibility to contamination of the wound from areas where there is high colonisation of bacteria.

Preparation for discharge is an ongoing process, which starts on admission, where information gathered relating to the child and family will influence and help predict subsequent care needs (Heath, 1998). Parents will often be extremely anxious about taking their child home, and will require detailed information relating to general caring skills, such as eating and drinking, bathing, resuming normal activities, specific care details, such as giving medications, wound care, and information about outpatients and return visits (Bailey and Caldwell, 1997). The number and range of healthcare professionals can often be overwhelming, so good communication within the team is essential. The information provided to the child and family must be accurate, consistent, delivered in an appropriate manner and documented (Bradford and Singer, 1991). Wherever possible, verbal advice should be supported with written advice. However, written advice is only of added value if it is clear, non-ambiguous, written in terms appropriate for the child and family, and in a language the family understands. Where the discharge is complex or specific care skills are required, a named worker should co-ordinate the process and there should be early referral and liaison with the community nursing team. It is vital that the family feels confident to take the child home into their care and is competent with any specialised care prior to discharge.

References

American Society of Anesthetists (ASA) Task Force (2002) Practice advisory for pre-anesthesia evaluation. *Anesthesiology* 96(2): 485–96

American Society of Anesthetists (ASA) Task Force (1999) Practice guidelines for preoperative fasting and the use of pharmacological agents to reduce the risks of pulmonary aspiration: application to healthy patients undergoing elective procedures. *Anesthesiology* 90(3): 896–905

Association of Anaesthetists (ASA) (2001) *Pre-operative Assessment and the Role of the Anaesthetist*. Association of Anaesthetists of Great Britain and Ireland, London, UK

Bailey R, Caldwell C (1997) Preparing parents for going home. *Paediatr Nurs* 9(4): 15–17

Baker JK, Borchers DA, Cochran DT *et al* (1989) Parent-child interaction model. In: Marriner T, ed. *Nursing Theorists and Their Work*, 2nd edn. Mosby, St Louis

Bates J (1994) Reducing fasting times in paediatric day care. *Nurs Times* 90(48): 38–39

Booker P (2000) Intravenous agents. In: Sumner E, Hatch DJ, eds. *Paediatric Anaesthesia*, 2nd edn. Edward Arnold, London

Boss S (2002) Expanding the perioperative role: the surgeon's assistant. *Br J Perioperat Nurs* 12(3): 105–13

Botti M, Hunt J (1994) The routine of post-operative observation. *Contemp Nurse* 3: 52–57

Bradford R, Singer H (1991) Support and information for parents. *Paediatr Nurs* 3(4): 18–20

Briggs M (1997) Principles of closed surgical wound care. *J Wound Care* 6(6): 288–92

Brown K, De Lima J, McEwan A *et al* (2000) Development and diseases in childhood. In: Sumner E, Hatch DJ, eds. *Paediatric Anaesthesia*, 2nd edn. Edward Arnold, London

Brown V (1997) The child in theatre: should parents be involved? *Br J Theare Nurs* 7(8): 5–7

Brown V (1995) Parents in recovery: parents and staff attitudes. *Paediatr Nurs* 7(7): 17–19

Brunt B, Gifford L, Hart D *et al* (1999) Designing Interdisciplinary documentation for the continuum of care. *J Nurs Qual Care* 14(1): 1–10

Burns LS (1997) Advances in Pediatric Anesthesia. *Nurs Clin N Am* 32(1): 45–71

Burroughs J, Hoffbrand B (1990) A critical look at nursing observation. *Postgrad Med J* **66**: 52–57

Casey A (1988) A partnership with child and family. *Senior Nurse* 8(4): 8–9

Cavell B (1979) Gastric emptying in preterm infants. *Acta Paediatrica Scand* **68**: 527–31

Cohen MM, Cameron CB, Duncan PG (1990) Pediatric anesthesia morbidity and mortality in the perioperative period. *Anesthes Analog* **70**: 160–67

Cowan T (1998) Peri-operative nursing. *Profess Nurse* **14**(1): 68–69

Currie L Harvey G (1997) *The Origins and Use of Care Pathways in the USA, Australia and the United Kingdom*. RCN Institute, Report No 5. Oxford Centre, Oxford

Department of Health (1993) *Calman report. Hospital Doctors: Training for the Future. Report on the Working Group of Specialist Medical Training*. HMSO, London

Department of Health (1991) *Welfare of Children and Young People in Hospital*. HMSO, London

Department of Health (1989) *The Children Act*. HMSO, London

Edlich RF, Jackson EM, Neal JG (2000) A scientific basis for choosing the technique of hair removal used prior to wound closure. *Emerg Nurs* **26**(2): 134–39

Eger EI (1994) New inhaled anesthetics. *Anesthesiol* **80**: 906–22

Emerson BM, Wrigley, SR, Newton M (1998). Preoperative fasting for paediatric anaesthesia. A survey of current practice. *Anaesthesia* **53**(4): 326–30

Ferrari LR, Rooney FM, Rockoff MA (1999) Pre-operative fasting practices in pediatrics. *Anesthesiol* **90**(4): 978–80

Fetzer SJ (2002) Reducing venipuncture and intravenous insertion pain with eutectic mixture of local anesthetic. *Nurs Res* **51**(2): 119–24

Fina DK, Lopas LJ, Stagnone JH *et al* (1997) Parental participation in the post-anesthesia care unit: fourteen years of progress at one hospital. *J Peri-anesthes Nurs* **12**(3): 152–62

Frayling IM, Addison GM, Chattergee K *et al* (1990) Methaemoglobinaemia in children treated with prilocaine-lignocaine cream. *Br Med J* **301**: 153–54

Goudsouzian N (2000) Relaxants in paediatric anaesthesia. In: Sumner E, Hatch DJ, eds. *Paediatric Anaesthesia*, 2nd edn. Edward Arnold, London

Gould D (2001) Clean surgical wounds: prevention of infection. *Nurs Stand* **15**(49): 45–52

Glasper A, Powell C (2000) First do no harm: parental exclusion from anaesthetic rooms. *Paediatr Nurs* **12**(4): 14–17

Hamilton JG (1995) Needle phobia: a neglected diagnosis. *Journal Fam Pract* **41**(2): 169–75

Hannallah RS, Epstein BS (1991) The pediatric patient. In: Wetchler BV, ed. *Anesthesia for Ambulatory Care*, 2nd edn. Lippincott, Philadelphia

Happs S (1994) Nursing: concepts, theories and models. In: Lindsay B, ed. *The Child and Family: Contemporary Nursing Issues in Child Health and Care*. Baillière Tindall, London

Heath S (1998) *Perioperative Care of the Child*. Mark Allen Publishing, Salisbury

Hogg C (1994) *Setting Standards for Children Undergoing Surgery*. Action for Sick Children, London

Horwitz J, Chawals W, Doski J et al (1998) Pediatric wound infections: a prospective multicentre study. *Annal Surg* **227**(4): 553–58

Howard R, Lloyd-Thomas A (2000) Pain management in children. In: Sumner E, Hatch DJ, eds. *Paediatric Anaesthesia*, 2nd edn. Edward Arnold, London

Imrie MM, Hall GM (1990) Body temperature and anaesthesia. *Br J Anaesthes* **64**: 346–54

Ingebo KR, Rayhorn NJ, Hecht RM et al (1997) Sedation in children: adequacy of two-hour fasting. *J Pediatrics* **1131**(1): 155–58

Kain ZN, Mayes LC, Wang SMD et al (2000) Parental presence and a premedicant for children undergoing surgery: a hierarchical study. *Anesthesioly* **92**(4): 939–46

Kain ZN, Mayes LC, Bell C et al (1997) Premedication in the United Stares; a status report. *Anesthesia Analgesia* **84**: 427–32

Kain ZN, Mayes LC, Caramico LA et al (1996) Parental presence during induction of anesthesia: a randomized control trial. *Anesthesiol* **84**(5): 1060–67

Kearney R, Mack C, Entwistle (1998) Withholding fluids from children undergoing day surgery reduces vomiting. *Paediatr Anesthesiol* **8**: 331–36

Kjønnisken I, Andersen BM, Søndenaa VG et al (2002) Preoperative hair removal—a systematic literature review. *AORN J* **75**(5): 928–36; 938; 940

Lawson RA, Smart NG, Gudgeon AC *et al* (1995) Evaluation of amethocaine gel for percutaneous analgesia before venous cannulation in children. *Br J Anaesthesia* **75**: 282–85

Leinonen T, Leino-Kilpi H (1999) Research in peri-operative nursing care. *J Clin Nurs* **8**(2): 123–38

Lerman J (1992) Surgical and patient factors involved in post-operative nausea and vomiting. *B J Anaesthesia* **69**: 24S–32S

Lowe C (1998) Care pathways: have they a place in the new National Health Service? *J Nurs Man* **6**(5): 303–306

Mangram AJ, Horan TC, Pearson ML *et al* (1999) Guideline for prevention of surgical site infection. *Am J Infect Contr* **27**(2): 97–132

McCormick AS, Spargo PM (1997) Parents in the anaesthetic room: a questionnaire survey of departments of anaesthesia. *Paediatric Anaesthesia* **6**: 187–93

McQuay HJ (1992) Pre-emptive analgesia. *Br J Anaesthesia* **69**: 1–3

Meakin G, Murat I (2000) Immediate preoperative preparation. In: Sumner E, Hatch DJ eds. *Paediatric Anaesthesia*, 2nd edn. Edward Arnold, London

Mirakhur RK (1991) Preanaesthetic medication; a survey of current usage. *J Roy Soc Med* **84**: 481–83

Munro J, Booth A, Nicholl J (1997) *Routine Preoperative Testing: A Systematic Review of the Evidence*. Health Technology Assessment, London: 1–12)

Nash PL, O'Malley M (1997) Streamlining the perioperative process. *Nurs Clin N Am* **32**(1): 141–51

National Confidential Enquiry into Perioperative Deaths, (1999) *Extremes of Age*. NCEPOD, London

National Health Service Management Executive (1991) *Junior Doctors: The New Deal*. NHSME, Leeds

Nicolson S, Schreiner M (1994) Feed the babies. *Anesthesia Analgesia* **79**: 407–409

Noble RR, Micheli AJ, Hensley MA *et al* (1997) Perioperative considerations for the pediatric patient: a developmental approach. *Nurs Clin N Am* **32**(10): 1–16

Norman L, Jones PL (1990) Complications of the use of EMLA. *British Journal of Anaesthesia* **64**: 403-406.

Norris AC (1998) Care pathways and the new NHS. *J Integr Care* **2**: 78–83

Nursing and Midwifery Council (2002) *Guidelines for Keeping Records and Record Keeping*. Nursing and Midwifery Council, London

Olsson G (2000) Monitoring in paediatric anaesthesia. In: Sumner E, Hatch DJ eds. *Paediatric Anaesthesia*, 2nd edn. Edward Arnold, London

Patel D, Meakin G (1997) Oral midazolam compared with diaze-pam-droperidol and trimeprazine as premedicants in children. *Paediatric Anaesthesia* 7: 287–93

Phillips S, Daborn AK, Hatch J (1994). Preoperative fasting for paediatric anaesthesia. *Br J Anaesthes* 73: 529–36

Pritchard MJ (2003) Malignant hyperthermia: clinical features and management. *Nurs Times* 99(23): 32–33

Rømsing J, Walther-Larsen S (1997) Peri-operative use of nonsteroidal anti-inflammatory drugs in children: analgesia efficacy and bleeding. *Anaesthesia* 52(7): 673–83

Roper N, Logan W, Tierney A (1996) *The Elements of Nursing: A Model for Nursing Based on a Model of Living*, 4th edn. Churchill Livingstone, Edinburgh

Roper N, Logan W, Tierney A (1980) *The Elements of Nursing: A Model for Nursing Based on a Model of Living*. Churchill Livingstone, Edinburgh

Royal College of Surgeons and Royal College of Anaesthetists (1990) *National Confidential Enquiry into Peripertaive Deaths 1989*. Royal College of Surgeons and Royal College of Anaesthetists, London

Royal College of Anaesthetists (2001) *Guidance on the Provision of Paediatric Anaesthetic Services*. Royal College of Anaesthetists, London

Rushforth H, Bliss A, Burge D *et al* (2000) Nurse-led pre-operative assessment: a study of appropriateness. *Paediatr Nurs* 12(5): 15–20

Rushforth H, Bliss A, Burge D *et al* (2000a) A pilot randomized control trial of medical versus nurse clerking for surgery. *Arch Dis Child* 83(3): 223–26

Rushforth H, Glasper EA (1999) Specialist nursing. Implications of nursing role expansion and professional practice. *Br J Nurs* 8(22): 1507–13

Schreiner M (1992) The pre-op fast: not quite so fast. *Contemp Pediatr* 6: 45–52

Sethi AK, Chatterji C, Bhargava SK *et al* (1999) Safe pre-operative fasting times after milk or clear fluid in children: a preliminary study using real-time ultrasound. *Anaesthesia* 54(1): 51–59

Small S (1996) Preoperative hair removal—a case report with implications for nursing. *J Clin Nurs* 5(2): 79–84

Smalley A (1999) Needle phobia. *Paediatr Nurs* 11(2): 17–20

Smith AF, Vallance H, Slater RM (1997) Shorter post-operative fluid fasts reduce post-operative emesis. *Br Med J* 314(7092): 1486

Smith F (1995) *Children's Nursing in Practice. The Nottingham Model.* Blackwell Science, Cambridge

Splinter WM, Schreiner MS (1999) Preoperative fasting in children. *Anesthesia Analgesia* 89: 80–89

Steward DJ (1982) Preterm infants are more prone to complications following minor surgery than are term infants. *Anesthesiol* 56: 304–306

Tait AR, Malviya S, Veopel-Lewis T *et al* (2001) Risk factors for perioperative adverse events in children with upper respiratory tract infections. *Anaesthesia* 95(2): 299–306

Tierney AJ (1998) Nursing models: extant or extinct? *J Adv Nurs* 28(10): 77–85.

United Kingdom Central Council for Nursing, Midwifery and Health Visiting (1992) *The Scope of Professional Practice.* UKCC, London

Walker I, Lockie J (2000) Basic techniques for anaesthesia. In: Sumner E, Hatch DJ eds. *Paediatric Anaesthesia*, 2nd edn. Edward Arnold, London

Watcha M (2000) The immediate recovery period. In: Sumner E, Hatch DJ eds. *Paediatric Anaesthesia*, 2nd edn. Edward Arnold, London

Welborn LG, Ramifrez N, Oh TH *et al* (1986) Postanesthetic apnea and periodic breathing in infants. *Anesthesiol* 65: 658–61

Wise J (1999) Perioperative nursing. *Profess Nurse* 15(1): 59–60

Wolf AR, Staddart PA, Murphy PJ *et al* (2002) Rapid skin anaesthesia using high velocity lignocaine particles: a prospective placebo controlled trial. *Arch Dis Child* 86(3): 309–12

Zeitz K, McCutcheon H (2002) Policies that drive the nursing practice of post-operative observation. *Int J Nurs Stud* 39: 831–39

FIVE

PRINCIPLES OF ACUTE PAIN MANAGEMENT

The International Association for the Study of Pain (IASP) introduced its first taxonomy of pain in 1979, which has subsequently been updated and defines pain as 'an unpleasant sensory and emotional experience associated with actual or potential tissue damage', (IASP, 1992: 2) and acute pain as 'a pain of recent onset of limited duration, which has useful purposes and is provoked by injury or disease' (IASP, 1992: 2). While less precise, McCaffery's (1968:1 11) earlier definition, 'pain is whatever the person experiencing it says it is, and existing whenever the person says it does' is popular because it reflects the individuality of the experience

Both definitions highlight the subjective and individual nature of pain, but may not be appropriate for children because their level of cognition will inevitably affect how they verbalise, localise and display a pain. Eland's (1990) studies indicate that the potential consequences of unrelieved acute pain include:

- Psychological consequences, such as recurrent nightmares or increased anxiety, and may influence decision-making in future healthcare interventions

- Bronchiectasis and atelectasis due to inadequate lung expansion

- Alkalosis due to increased respiratory rate and shallow breathing

- Chest infection due to increased secretions accumulating from inadequate cough and lack of spontaneous movement

- Rapid respirations, increased heart rate, increased perspiration and increased metabolic rate that will increase fluid losses.

All have the potential to delay and complicate the recovery of the child who has undergone a surgical procedure. Pain management is a vital component of the care of a child requiring the surgery. This chapter will:

- Provide an overview of the neurophysiology of pain in order to understand the principles of pain management
- Outline the myths surrounding children's perception of pain
- Describe pain assessment
- Outline principles of pain management
- Discuss ways of improving pain services for children.

5.1 Overview of pain physiology

There are many interconnections within the central nervous system that come into play following initiation of a nerve impulse in response to a painful stimulus, which are potential sites for enhancing or inhibiting impulse. A noxious stimulus, which creates a nerve impulse to be triggered, only becomes perceived as 'pain' when the sensation reaches conscious levels, resulting in a unique and specific experience for each individual. The physiology of pain has been described as a four-stage process: transduction, transmission, perception and modulation (Hawthorn and Redmond, 1998) (*Figure 5.1a*).

Transduction

Transduction is the detection of a painful stimulus by nociceptive receptors. Nociceptors are free nerve endings (branch ends of dendrites of certain sensory neurons) that respond to noxious stimuli (Heuther and Leo, 2002). Nociceptors are found in practically every tissue of the body and are especially numerous in skin and muscle (Heuther and Leo, 2002). They can be activated by a variety of stimuli, either internal or external. Stimuli include chemical mediators of local cell damage (such as bradykinins, serotonin and prostaglandins or external chemi-

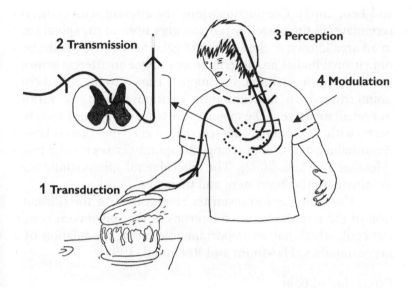

2 Transmission

3 Perception

4 Modulation

1 Transduction

Figure 5.1a: Schematic representation of the stages of pain pathways: transduction, transmission, perception and modulation

cals), electrical, thermal radiation and mechanical forces (for example tissue swelling or external pressure). Most nociceptors are polymodal and respond to other stimuli, such as touch, pressure, heat and cold (Heuther and Leo, 2002). If these sensations reach a certain threshold, they can be perceived as a painful sensation.

Transmission

Transmission is the process by which nociceptors relay information to the central nervous system (Hawthorn and Redmond, 1998). Sensory (afferent) nerve fibres conduct impulses from nociceptors to the spinal cord. In relation to pain, sensory nerve fibres are either Aδ fibres (large myelinated fibres with fast impulse speeds, usually located in cutaneous tissues, producing sensations which are often well defined, such as those associated with acute pain) or C fibres (non-myelinated and having a smaller diameter, thus a slower response, often associated with chronic pain where sensations may be diffuse and dull) (Heuther and Leo, 2002). Conduction along the afferent sensory nerves terminates in the posterior (dorsal) grey horn of the spinal cord in an area known as the substantia gelatinosa (SG), a collection of neuronal bodies and interneurones. Once an afferent sensory nerve has been activated, the impulse travels to the spinal cord uninterrupted. In the substantia gelatinosa there are various intermediate nerves. The majority cross the spinal cord and connect with ascending nerves to form the anterolateral spinothalmic tract, connecting the spinal cord with the brain (Heuther and Leo, 2002). The anterolateral spinothalmic tract terminates in the brain stem and thalamus.

The main neurotransmitter responsible for the transmission of the impulse between neurons in the spinal cord is substance P, which has an important role in the modulation of a nerve impulses (Hawthorn and Redmond, 1998).

Perception of pain

Perception of pain occurs when the brain receives a nerve stimulus, which is interpreted as a painful sensation (Hawthorn and Redmond, 1998). Although there does not appear to be a specific pain centre within the brain, there are specific regions of the brain that are actively involved in perceiving stimuli as a painful sensation and co-ordinating a response to the stimuli. Areas of particular importance are the postcentral gyrus, reticular formation, pons, limbic system, midbrain, thalamus and sensory cortex (Heuther and Leo, 2002). All nerves transmitting impulses from nociceptors eventually synapse in the thalamus. From here nerve pathways transcend to the sensory cortex in the cerebral hemispheres. This is where knowledge, previous experience, and cultural influences probably exert their effects upon the perception of pain. Axons from the spinothalamic tract also connect with the medulla, hypothalamus and limbic system before reaching the thalamus (Heuther and Leo, 2002). It is thought that these pathways and other sensory stimuli help co-ordination of the autonomic system's response; for example, moving away from a dangerous situation.

The reticular formation consists of a complex matrix of nerve cells within the brain stem that have many interconnections, including nerve fibres from the spinal cord to the thalamus and vice versa, and is thought to play an important part in modulation of the pain experience (Hawthorn and Redmond, 1998). The limbic system consists of a number of important nuclei deep within the brain, with complex actions. It is thought to be the site where primitive responses are initiated and co-ordinates responses to higher brain thought processes (Longstaff, 2000). The limbic system may influence the immediate actions taken by the body and may account for the psychological, emotional and behavioural response to pain.

Modulation

Various theories have been postulated to explain the physiological and psychological processes involved in the pain experience and the modulation of pain pathways, in an attempt to explain the uniqueness of the experience (Hawthorn and Redmond, 1998). There are probably several mechanisms that contribute to the modulation process. The body contains naturally-occurring substances, such as neuropeptides, that have a modulation effect on pain pathways (Heuther and Leo, 2002). For example, one of the properties of substance P is to enhance the transmission of a stimulus by speeding up the reaction at synapses. Preventing the action of substance P will potentially have an analgesic effect. Endogenous opioids (enkephalins and endorphins), found predominantly in the thalamus, hypothalamus, specific areas of the limbic system and spinal cord, bind with opioid receptor sites, blocking the action of substance P and other excitatory neurotransmitters (Heuther and Leo, 2002). In addition, endogenous opioids act by blocking the release of substance P at nerve receptor sites.

In an attempt to explain the integration of physiological and psychological dimension of pain, Wall and Melzack (1989) proposed the 'gate control pain theory' and, although there are other theories, it is the most widely accepted. The theory proposes that there is a 'gating mechanism' in the dorsal horn of the spinal cord through which peripheral information passes. The degree to which the 'gate' is opened or closed will determine the degree of the pain perception. The 'gating mechanism' consists of two types of cells; SG cells (which have an inhibitory effect) and T cells (which have an activation effect). There appears to be two interactive systems that influence the 'gating' mechanism.

The first is competitive peripheral input. When peripheral nerve impulses from nociceptor stimulation arrive at the dorsal horn and reach a critical level, T cells are activated, the 'gate' opens, allowing information to flow up to the thalamus and to the sensory cortex, resulting in the perception of pain (Wall and Melzack, 1989) (*Figure 5.1b*). However, there are situations where the 'gate' can remain closed despite stimulation by a nerve impulse originating from a nociceptor; for example, activation of the SG cells from competing non-painful peripheral nerve input (Wall and Melzack, 1989). The classic example of this competitive nerve input explains the pain inhibition that occurs when 'mummy rubs it better'. A kick on the knee would activate nociceptors and, if the stimulus was large enough, a nerve impulse would be initiated, arriving in the spinal cord and activating T cells. The 'gate' would open and allow interconnections to be made via the spinal cord to the brain. However, if the knee is vigorously rubbed non-painful sensory fibres would be activated and transmission of a nerve impulse would occur in these large diameter fibres, which stimulate the SG cells. In this situation, the nociceptor and pressure sensory stimulation are competing to open or close the 'gate'; eventually, the stronger impulse will dominate.

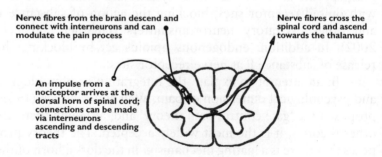

Nerve fibres from the brain descend and connect with interneurons and can modulate the pain process

Nerve fibres cross the spinal cord and ascend towards the thalamus

An impulse from a nociceptor arrives at the dorsal horn of spinal cord; connections can be made via interneurons ascending and descending tracts

Figure 5.1b: Spinal cord pathways

The second type of modulation at the dorsal horn is the influence of the descending nerves from the brain; for example, the corticospinal and reticulospinal tracts, descending tracts that have the potential to stimulate the SG cells or the T cells, thus to open or close the gate (Wall and Melzack, 1989) (*Figure 5.1b*). In addition, the reticular formation has opioid receptors that can modulate the pain response.

5.2 Perception of pain in children; myths and misconceptions

Many children in hospital suffer unnecessary pain (Twycross, 1998a) because of inadequate recognition and, consequently, inadequate management of their pain (Eland and Anderson, 1977; Mather and Mackie, 1983; McIlvaine, 1989; Schechter *et al*, 1986; Wills, 2002). Initially, the lack of an evidence-base upon which to build practice contributed to poor pain management in children (Twycross, 2002; 1998a). However, since the mid 1980s, there has been a proliferation of published research relating to pain management in children, which, unfortunately, does not appear to have resulted in a change or improvement in practice (Stevens and Koren, 1998). Cummings *et al*'s (1996) study indicated that many children still experience significant pain during hospital admission and, more recently, Byrne *et al*'s (2001) study suggest that nurses denied the reality of pain experienced by children in an attempt to protect themselves from emotional stress, which compromised the provision of effective pain management.

Healthcare professionals have many myths and misconceptions in relation to the pain experience and management of pain in children, including:

- Infants cannot feel pain because of an immature nervous system
- Children do not feel as much pain as adults
- Narcotic use is dangerous in children
- Active children cannot be in pain

- Sleeping children cannot be in pain
- Children engaged in play cannot be in pain
- Pain results in children crying
- Children always tell the truth about their pain
- Injections are not painful
- Giving a child an injection results in hostility towards the carer.

(Burr, 1993; Eland, 1990)

Recent research suggests that many of these original misconceptions relating to children's pain still exist. Simons *et al*'s (2001) study identified parents who were concerned about nurses' attitudes towards their child's pain; for example, if a child had not voiced any concern, then he/she must not be in pain, and parents not being believed when expressing concerns about their child's pain, with the majority of parents dissatisfied with their child's pain management. Byrne *et al*'s (2001) study found that nurses displayed many negative responses to a child's needs, such as viewing the child's pain as unreal, unwarranted and for some children, not deserving help. Both studies indicate that nurses do not appear to embody the principles of caring for children and there are many negative attitudes towards pain management.

Factors that affect nurses' perceptions of pain in children, include:

- Nurses who have experiences of their own child experiencing pain are more aware of the pain needs of children
- The type of unit influences analgesia choices, with critical care units using opioids more frequently
- The priority given to pain management
- Highly educated nurses used higher doses of analgesia
- The workload of nurses influenced pain interventions
- Cultural differences between nurses and children and their families were a barrier to providing adequate pain management

- Attitudes of staff
- The child's age, with the non-verbal child receiving less analgesia
- Disease process and type of treatments
- Child's temperament, expression and behaviours.

(Twycross, 2002a; 2001)

The inability of young children to verbalise their needs and the lack of valid and reliable assessment tools across the age spectrum compound the difficulties for staff trying to relieve children's pain (Jackson, 1995). Furthermore, young children adopt many coping strategies, such as avoiding interactions, resisting behaviours and self-protection behaviours, which to the uninformed could lead to misinterpreting the child's needs (Woodgate and Kristjanson, 1995).

Buckingham (1993) advocates working within a developmental framework and, for the pre-verbal child, close observation of his/her behavioural responses. In order to understand a child's perception of pain, it is essential that healthcare professionals are knowledgeable about the physiological differences between children and adults, and relate a child's developmental stage to age-specific concepts of pain and illness-behaviours. The physiological differences between a child and an adult are not logically applied when considering the child's ability to perceive and interpret pain. For example, peripheral nerve myelination is not complete until about the third year of life (Volpe, 1981) and was often used to rationalise the concept that neonates were unable to perceive pain. This is obviously an inappropriate belief as myelination only affects the speed of a response and does not act as an inhibitor. The neonate may also be able to compensate for lack of myelination, as there are also other factors that contribute to the speed of an impulse, such as the length of nerve axon, the diameter of nerve and temperature. In fact, due to the size of the neonate and increased metabolic rate, this may result in a faster response. By 28 weeks of gestation, active and effective nociceptors and ascending pain transmission pathways are present, indicating that the neonate has the ability to sense painful stimuli and transmit nerve impulses to the central nervous system (Fitzgerald and Beggs, 2001). Conversely, although only demonstrated in animal studies, descending tracts do develop later in the maturation process (Fitzgerald and Koltzenburg, 1986); therefore, the neonate, in addition to lacking experience, will not have an inhibitory feedback system, resulting in an inability to modify the intensity of pain experience.

There is no evidence to support the misconception that opioid use is more dangerous in children than adults. In fact the evidence reviewed by Walco *et al* (1994) suggests that although the potential risks with opioid use, such as respiratory depression or arrest, are real, the incidence in children is no greater than adults and may well be less. Concerns relating to addiction are negligible in adults and virtually non-existent in children (Walco *et al*, 1994). The level of a child's activity seems to cause confusion. Pain is an extremely discrete response and, depending upon the cause and duration of the pain, the level of activity will be individual to each child. A child who is actively verbalising through shouting or crying may alert healthcare professionals that there is an unmet need. However, pain can result in exhaustive sleep (Hawley, 1984), and because many children will attempt distraction techniques through play in order to cope with distress (Woodgate and Kristjanson, 1995), these children also have unmet needs.

There may be many reasons for a child not to tell the truth about his/her pain, such as fear of the cause of the pain, a belief that it is a punishment for wrong-doing, therefore must be endured, and fear of the consequences, particularly injections (Mather and Mackie, 1983). Intra-muscular injections have been described by children as the worst hurt they have ever experienced (Eland, 1981). In addition to the misconceptions relating to the interpretation of physiological differences between children and adults, a child's individual perception of the cause and effect of pain will be influenced by many factors, including: their age, cognitive and linguistic abilities, experience, personality, family and cultural beliefs. Younger children will have much fewer experiences to draw upon and will be less likely to have the ability to anticipate the outcome of the pain and decide how to plan effective coping strategies. This heightened anxiety may intensify the perception of pain.

Children between four and 12 years are the most frequently studied age group in relation to all aspects of pain management, probably due to the fact that their linguistic skills are sufficient to self-report their pain levels, a variety of pain tools have been demonstrated to be reliable with this age group, and the presence of resident parents will enable consent to be obtained to participate in research (Maikler, 1998). Linguistic barriers need considering; for example, the word 'pain' and 'hurt' may be entirely absent from a young child's vocabulary (Carter *et al*, 2002; Thompson and Varni, 1986). In general, there is limited primary research relating to the developmental stage of a child and his/her perceptions of, and response to, pain. Exceptions include work by Hurley and Whelan (1988) and Woodgate and Kristjanson (1995). Piaget's (1952) (*Appendix I*) stages of cognitive development appear to be the most frequently used when describing how a child's perception of pain changes through maturation (Gaffney *et al*, 2003; Hurley and Whelan, 1988; Thompson and Varni, 1986; Twycross, 1998a). *Table 5.2a* provides examples of how a child may express/present with pain, and the implications for practice.

Table 5.2a: Age-specific perceptions of pain in children and implications for practice (adapted from Gaffney *et al*, 2003; Twycross, 1998)

Piaget's stage of development	Perception/presentation of pain	Implications for practice
Sensorimotor (0–2 years)	In this age group, pain will be a physical experience and primarily be expressed by changes in behaviours, such as restlessness, irritability, tense, abnormal crying/grizzling/screaming, abnormal posture/movements.	Understanding the normal activities and behaviours for each individual child and comparing these to those presented during illness is paramount. Excellent observations skills are necessary, particularly in relation to interpreting verbal sounds/words, facial expression and body language.
Pre-operational (2–7 years)	Again, pain is primarily perceived as a physical experience, with an inability to distinguish between the cause of pain and its effect. Pain is often perceived as a result of their own behaviour; for example, as a punishment for a wrongdoing. However, pain may also be perceived as the responsibility of someone else and the child may believe magical acts can remove the pain. Many express behaviours similar to those of infants. Increased ability to verbalise needs will correlate to language skills developments.	Carers must be aware that the child may be aggressive when offered help and will not understand the connection between treatment and pain relief. Allowing the child to express his/her feelings is important; encourage the child to describe the pain in his/her own language. Much reassurance is needed to explain pain is not a punishment. Family input is vital; however, parents may not have experienced their child in pain and not understand the change in behaviours. Guidance relating to comforting their child and distraction techniques will be necessary.
Concrete operational (7–12 years)	There is more understanding and perception of the physical properties of pain and can now relate pain to body parts. Fear about the consequence of pain and damage to the body are great; vivid imagination can lead to fears of total body destruction. Towards the end of this period, some rational thinking develops. Pain concepts beginning to form and the child can describe effects that influence pain—the 'if' and 'when' scenarios.	The child needs clear explanations about cause of pain and treatments, and opportunity to discuss fears and beliefs and reassurance should be given relating to body destruction.
Formal operational (12 years and older)	There are the beginnings of depth of understanding, but these may not be consistent due to limited life experiences and therefore the child may imagine sinister consequences of the pain.	Adolescents need clear explanations about causes of pain and treatments, and opportunity to discuss fears and beliefs about the potential impact of the pain.

5.3 Assessment of pain in children

Pain management practices in children do not appear to be based upon a systematic assessment of the child, analgesia does not appear to be administered consistently to children, and non-pharmacological interventions are rarely considered (Jacob and Puntillo, 1999). 'Effective pain management is fundamentally linked to effective assessment' (Carter, 1994: 39), and serves two main purposes: to ensure interventions are appropriate and to evaluate the effectiveness of interventions. The clinical assessment of pain should be based upon the four components of pathology, child behaviours, verbalisation and assessment tools. In addition, physiological changes will occur in episodes of acute pain (Eland, 1990). These components are similar to the QUESTT framework developed for assessing pain in children (Baker and Wong, 1987), which involves Questioning the child, Using a pain rating scale, Evaluating behaviours and physiological changes, Securing family involvement, Taking the cause of the pain into account, Taking action and evaluating response.

Question the child and secure family involvement

Ideally, assessment should occur before the child experiences pain. In an acute situation, it may not be possible to perform a detailed pain assessment immediately, but this should not cause a delay in providing analgesia. An effective pain assessment is a crucial component of pre-operative care for all children undergoing elective surgery. The child and family should be questioned about the child's previous experiences of pain, any specific behaviours the child may display which could indicate the presence of pain, the child's understanding of pain, and the child's developmental stage. There needs to be an understanding of the family's attitudes towards pain, which should include the potential influence of cultural, religious and spiritual beliefs. This information, in conjunction with knowledge of the type of surgery and the predicted intensity of post-operative pain, will enable healthcare professionals to discuss and plan with the child and family the type and mode of delivery of post-operative analgesia. Unfortunately, healthcare professionals often view the family as having a passive role in relation to the management of the child's pain (Simons *et al*, 2001). Where possible, the child should be involved in deciding the pain assessment tool, and the child and family should have a detailed explanation about its use.

Pain assessment tools

Despite the development of a range of pain assessment tools for the use in children, it has been suggested that many are not reliable and valid (Jackson, 1995; Taylor, 1998; Thompson and Varni, 1986), which may be due to difficulties in producing a tool that is practical, versatile and free from individual bias. However in 1999, the Royal College of Nursing (UK) produced clinical practice guidelines relating to the recognition and assessment of acute pain in children. Despite difficulties with assessment tools, the Royal College of Nursing recommended their use because of evidence suggesting children receive more analgesia and therefore a reduction in pain when tools are used. The guidelines also recommended that self-report tools for those children who can communicate are the 'gold standard', because a child's own subjective account is the single most reliable indicator of the intensity of pain. Concepts and language associated with pain probably begin at about eight years of age (La Fleur and Raway, 1999), which have implications for the format of self- report tools. Verbal descriptors of pain may be inappropriate below this age. Without the ability to directly measure 'pain', assessment tools are a vital component of the assessment process. Wood (2002) suggests that uni-dimensional tools (measuring one aspect of the pain experience, for example, pain intensity) are fairly accurate, easy to understand and are quick to use. This makes them ideal for use in acute and post-operative situations. Examples of uni-dimensional tools include: visual analogue scales, verbal rating scales, numerical rating scale, graphical rating scales, verbal descriptor scales, behaviour rating scales, body diagrams and picture scales. The Royal College of Nursing (1999) clinical practice guidelines provide detailed evaluation of 25 types of pain assessment tools across the age spectrum in children. Examples include:

- *Infants and toddlers* (pre-verbal)

  Children unable to verbalise will be unable to use a self-report assessment tool. The range of tools for assessing pain in this group of children includes: objective pain scale, cries, CHEOPS (Children's Hospital of Eastern Ontario Pain Scale) and LIDS (Liverpool Infant Distress Score) and, specifically for use in the premature infant, are the NFCS (Neonatal Facial Coding System) and PIPP (Premature Infant Pain Profile) tools (Royal College of Nursing, 1999). These tools rely upon the assessor's interpretation of the child's behaviour and make an assumption about the presence and nature of 'pain'. This can place considerable demands on healthcare professionals in distinguishing between normal behaviours and pain behaviours (Carter, 1994). In addition, many of the assessment tools for this age range are complex and complicated to use (Royal College of Nursing, 1999), which is a disadvantage in busy clinical areas. Behaviour pain assessment tools incorporate variables related to facial expression, crying and body posture aspects (*Figure 5.3a*).

Score	Appearance/behaviours
0	Laughing, smiling, contented Gurgling, cooing, chatting Actively playing, contented/restful sleep
I	Distracts easily Articulating pain, moaning, complaining in general Grimaces on movement
2	Able to distract for short periods only Withdrawn, miserable Touching area of body repeatedly, uncomfortable, restless
3	Difficult to distract Miserable, moaning, crying Irritable, sensitive to handling, guarding
4	Unable to distract Screaming, aggressive, persistently grimacing Abnormally still, body rigid/tense position, sleep exhausted

Figure 5.3a: Relationship between infant appearance/behaviours and pain score

- *Young children*

  A variety of pictorial scales have been designed for use with young children; probably the most familiar are Wong and Baker's (1988) and Bieri *et al's* (1990) faces pain scales, consisting of a series of six and seven faces respectively, expressing various emotions which correlate to pain intensity. The Royal College of Nursing (1999) suggests five faces on a scale of 0–4. Faces scales are easy to use and user friendly; however, younger children tend to choose faces at the extremities of the scale (Royal College of Nursing, 1999). There is a need to explain the link between the faces and pain because, for some children, this will not be self-evident (Taylor, 1998) and they may confuse it with a 'happiness' measure (Royal College of Nursing, 1999). They are generally suitable for three to seven years of age. *Figure 5.3b* illustrates a five-face scale.

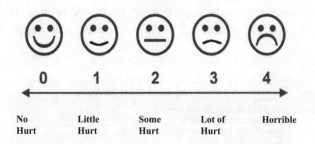

Figure 5.3b: Example of a faces pain scale and pain score

  Other pain assessment tools suitable for this age group include poker chip tool, colour scales and Oucher scales (Royal College of Nursing, 1999).

- *Older children*

  Visual analogue scales consist of a vertical line, usually 10cm, with the words 'no pain at all' and 'worst possible pain' written at opposite ends of the line (Taylor, 1998) (*Figure 5.3c*), and measures the magnitude of the pain. The child is asked to mark on the line the level of their pain. Although the scale can be used with children where language is limited (the child's own words can be substituted), the child must have the ability to think abstractly in order to translate the pain experience to a visual line. It is therefore inappropriate for pre-operational children. The advantages of the visual analogue scale is freedom for the child to express the pain at the exact level he/she is experiencing. A major drawback occurs once the visual analogue scale has been used in that, without a numerical value, using the tool in conjunction with an analgesic ladder (*Figure 5.4a*) necessitates healthcare professionals making judgements about the position of the mark and linking this to the appropriate intervention.

No pain at all — **worst possible pain**

Figure 5.3c: Example of a visual analogue scale

Verbal rating scales are a similar design to the visual analogue scale; however, there is a list of adjectives, such as 'no pain', 'mild pain', 'moderate pain', 'severe pain', 'very severe pain' along the line; these may be associated with a numerical value.

Numerical rating scales are again similar tools, but the line is divided into a scale usually, 1 to 10.

The choice of tool will depend upon the clinical setting and type of pain. Pain tools should be based upon the following criteria: ratio scaling properties, relatively free from individual practitioner bias, provide immediate and accurate information, reliable and generalisable, sensitive to changes in pain intensity, simple and easy to use (Schofield, 1995). It is important to use a pain assessment tool appropriate to the child's developmental stage, personality and condition (Royal College of Nursing, 1999). No one tool will 'fit' all.

It is vital to consider individual requirements for the child with special needs, because less able and inarticulate children may receive sub-standard care and less analgesia than their able counterparts (Twycross *et al*, 1999). Parents of children with special needs often feel isolated when dealing with their child's pain (Carter *et al*, 2002a). Although for many of these children, pain has become an intrinsic part of the child's life, when additional factors contribute or change this normal tolerance, parents need guidance from healthcare professionals in relation to pain assessment and strategies to relieve pain (Carter *et al*, 2002a). Parents often devise their own frameworks for assessing their child's pain, which should be incorporated into nursing care plans. None of the parents involved in Carter *et al*'s (2002a) study had received any educational input relating to pain management from healthcare professionals.

Pain assessment tools are an integral aspect of the overall pain strategies used in clinical areas and it is important that they complement these strategies (*Section 5.4*).

Evaluating behaviours and physiological changes

Changes in a child's behaviour, appearance, activity and physiological variables may indicate a change in pain intensity (Carter, 1994; Royal College of Nursing, 1999; Tatman and Johnson, 1998; Taylor, 1998). Behavioural tools have already been described and have become an important component in the assessment of the child who is unable to use self-report tools (Carter, 1994). Alterations in behaviours, such as a child becoming restless, having sleep disturbances, who cannot be distracted easily, shortened attention span and refusal to eat, may indicate pain (Eland, 1990). Behavioural assessment tools should be used cautiously and may assess a range of behavioural responses, for example distress, hunger and isolation from parents (Carter, 1994). In the verbal child, behavioural assessment should be used in conjunction with a self-report tool.

Physiological changes that may occur as a result of pain include: elevation of heart rate, decreased oxygen saturation levels, increased respiratory rate, slight increase in blood pressure and increased palmar sweating (Carter, 1994). Physiological measures should only be used in addition to assessment tools, because the evidence available to support changes in physiological parameters alone, which can be directly attributable to a pain response, are generally weak and inconsistent (Royal College of Nursing, 1999). Although physiological changes may be related to pain, they may also be due to many other factors, such as infection, change in haemodynamic status, trauma and, in fact, anything that triggers a stress response (Eland, 1990). In addition, over-reliance of physiological changes could result in an underestimation of the level of pain, primarily because the body's acute response to pain cannot be maintained.

The final components of the QUESTT (Baker and Wong, 1987) framework—take action and evaluate response—will be discussed in the next section.

5.4 Methods of pain control in children

It is essential that post-operative pain is managed promptly and efficiently in order to reduce the distress of the child and improve the outcome of surgery. Providing effective pain management is not only an integral component of nursing care (Nursing and Midwifery Council, 2001), but also one of the basic rights for all children, recognised by the United Nations Convention on the Rights of the Child (Newell, 1991). Ensuring effective pain management is dependent upon successful multidisciplinary working (Mackintosh and Bowles, 2000), with clear roles and responsibilities and a pain management plan for each individual child (Carr, 1997), working in collaboration with the child and family (Royal College of Nursing, 1999; Simons *et al*, 2001). Despite the increased use of pain assessment tools, there is little evidence to support the relationship between the assessment, interventions and subsequent evaluations of pain because of a lack of understanding of the problem-solving cycle involved in pain management (Carr, 1997). Although nurses may be efficient at administering analgesic drugs, the overall management of pain in children is poor, with lack of systematically undertaken assessments and little consideration for non-pharmacological interventions (Twycross, 2002). An integral part of the strategies for managing pain in children will involve choosing the best pain control interventions. Multi-modal interventions are important, but in the management of acute pain, non-pharmacological interventions should be used only as an adjunct to pharmacological agents (Wood, 2002a).

Pharmacological interventions

The type of drug intervention will depend upon several factors: the pain assessment, cause of the pain, the therapeutic action of the drug, intensity and location of the pain, and the individual child's needs (Broadbent, 2000). An analgesic ladder, although initially developed by the World Health Organization (1998) for chronic cancer pain, is a useful concept in that drugs of similar potency can be grouped together (*Figure 5.4a*). The ladder is used in a stepwise approach in that if a drug is ineffective, it is

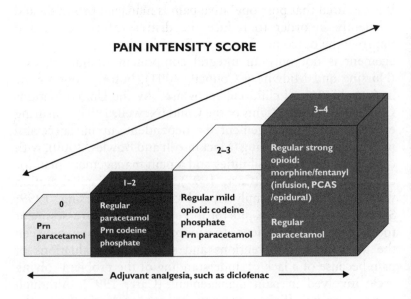

PAIN INTENSITY SCORE

| 0 | 1–2 | 2–3 | 3–4 |

Prn paracetamol

Regular paracetamol
Prn codeine phosphate

Regular mild opioid: codeine phosphate
Prn paracetamol

Regular strong opioid: morphine/fentanyl (infusion, PCAS /epidural)

Regular paracetamol

◄———— Adjuvant analgesia, such as diclofenac ————►

Figure 5.4a: An example of an analgesic ladder

important to move to the group of drugs on the next rung of the ladder, which may have the desired effect. It is important to start on the correct rung of the ladder (Carter, 1994). Particularly useful adjunctive therapies include: non-steroidal anti-inflammatory drugs, such as diclofenac, and muscle relaxants, such as baclofen.

An analgesic ladder should simplify and guide in the prescription of analgesia, but be flexible and sensitive enough to meet a child's individual needs. This can be achieved by having four drug choices that have a range of actions and potencies, such as paracetamol, diclofenac, codeine phosphate and morphine (Moriarty, 1998).

Paracetamol is the most commonly prescribed analgesic in children (Carter, 1994). Despite this, it is often used inappropriately (Moriarty, 1998) and is only really appropriate for mild pain or as an adjunct to more potent analgesics. Although its exact mode of action is unknown, paracetamol is thought to act by inhibiting prostaglandin synthesis in the brain. It, therefore, probably impairs the perception of pain. There is little evidence as to the effectiveness of combining analgesics, but a non-steroidal anti-inflammatory drug, such as diclofenac given as an adjuvant with regular paracetamol, can often provide effective analgesia (National Prescribing Centre, 2000). Oral paracetamol is dependent on effective gastrointestinal functioning, so is inappropriate following gastrointestinal surgery until gut motility returns. The increasing use of paracetamol fastmelts, which dissolve on the tongue, are improving the analgesics options for children nil by mouth. Paracetamol is available and effective in a suppository format, but this mode of delivery may be unacceptable to some children and their wishes should be respected. Care must be taken not to exceed the recommended maximum daily dose, calculated on body weight, due to potential liver damage. This is an important consideration if paracetamol is given on discharge, as many over-the-counter preparations (for colds and influenza) contain paracetamol and a number of trade names could be misleading for parents (Broadbent, 2000).

Diclofenac is a non-steroidal anti-inflammatory drug with analgesic, anti-inflammatory and antipyretic properties. Like all non-steroidal anti-inflammatory drugs, diclofenac acts by inhibiting prostaglandin synthesis and is thought to act predominantly peripherally by antagonising the effect of prostaglandins at nociceptor receptor sites. However, inhibition of prostaglandins can cause decreased platelet activity, increased risk of gastrointestinal bleeding and decreased renal blood flow, but side-effects appear to be less common in children (Moriarty, 1998). Non-steroidal anti-inflammatories are contraindicated if there is a renal impairment, hypovolaemia, low platelets or tendency to bleed, liver disease, and gastric ulceration. They are also contraindicated in children under six months, immuno-compromised children, and should be used with caution in children with asthma (may increase symptoms) (Moriarty, 1998). Diclofenac is available in a range of oral forms including a suspension (making it suitable for small doses), and in suppository form; again dosage will need to be calculated on body weight. It is useful for mild to moderate pain and as an adjunct to other analgesics.

Opioid analgesics are used for moderate to severe pain. Opiods act on specific opioid receptors in the central nervous system (and probably within the peripheral nervous system), inhibiting impulses reaching areas of the brain, such as the reticular formation, limbic system, thalamus and sensory cortex where pain is perceived; in addition, opioids have a sedative effect (Longstaff, 2000). Codeine phosphate is a weak opioid, effective at relieving mild to moderate pain, and is best used in conjunction with diclofenac and paracetamol (Moriarty, 1998). Codeine phosphate is available in a wide range of oral, suppository and injectable forms. Intramuscular injection only is recommended because intravenous injection results in apnoea and severe hypotension (Yaster and Deshpande, 1988). A major limiting factor with codeine phosphate is its constipating effect.

Despite advances in analgesics, morphine sulphate is still the 'gold standard opioid' against which all others drugs are compared and is the drug of choice in severe pain (Moriarty, 1998). Morphine is available in a wide range of preparations and can be given orally, rectally, intramuscularly, subcutaneously and intravenously. In addition, the increased recognition that acute pain requirements are ongoing has resulted in the development of continuous infusion systems for intravenous routes (Bray *et al*, 1986). The choice of route and method of administration will depend upon many factors, including:

- The pain severity score

- Reasons or cause of pain, for example, trauma, surgery, predicted duration of acute pain

- The child's cognitive level and abilities; this is particularly important when considering patient-controlled analgesia systems

- Physical status; for example, oral medication is not suitable if a child is vomiting or has impaired gut motility, subcutaneous may not be suitable if there is poor tissue perfusion, and intravenous administration may not be appropriate if venous access is problematic

- Ability to monitor the child

- Time available to prepare the child and family; this is particularly important in patient-controlled analgesia systems

- Support available from anaesthetic services/pain services

- Local practice, policies and guidelines.

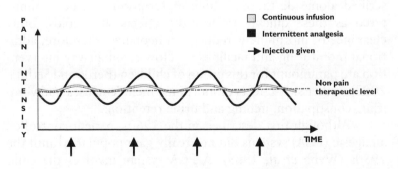

Figure 5.4b: Continuous infusion v intermittent intramuscular injections

Children's fear of injections (Eland, 1981; Mather and Mackie, 1983) and the peaks and troughs associated with intermittent intramuscular injections (Bray *et al*, 1986; Maikler, 1998) (*Figure 5.4b*) makes their use inappropriate in children.

Continuous intravenous morphine infusions have been used in the management of post-operative pain following major surgery in children since the early 1980s (Bray *et al*, 1986; Bray, 1983) because of their ability to produce more consistent analgesia levels and the facility to add bolus doses as required. Despite successful use over the past two decades, with research supporting its efficacy and safety in older children (Berde and Sethna, 2002), there are still misconceptions about the use of opioids in children (Broadbent, 2000). Unfounded over-estimation of potential risks leads to an underestimation of the potential harm of pain, and the under-medication of children (Walco *et al*, 1994). Excessive sedation and respiratory depression are undesirable side-effects of morphine and remain a concern because of the potential for eventual respiratory arrest. However, the risk is minimal if weight-related doses are used and children are appropriately monitored (Walco *et al*, 1994). In addition, severe consequences, such as respiratory arrest, can be prevented because respiratory slowing occurs well before severe respiratory depression. Appropriate interventions, such as slowing or stopping the infusion, can be implemented and, if necessary, antidotes such as naloxone, which should always be prescribed alongside the morphine prescription, can be administered as these quickly reverse the effects of opioids. Body clearance of morphine is reduced in neonates; therefore, additional monitoring and facilities to allow rapid airway intervention are paramount for this group of children (Berde and Sethna, 2002). Other side-effects of morphine include nausea and vomiting, constipation, itching and urine retention.

Although first described in the 1960s, patient-controlled analgesic (PCA) systems did not really gain popularity until the 1980s (Webb *et al*, 1989). A PCA system involves the child administering a bolus dose of analgesia (usually morphine intravenously) to coincide with any pain experienced. As with continuous morphine infusions, adult PCA regimes do not translate into paediatric practice (Moriarty, 1998) because of the need to use weight-related doses and the preference to use a concurrent reduced dose background infusion (Berde *et al*, 1991), which appears to improve pain management in children. The use of PCA has been found to be particularly valuable in children 11–18 years of age, and is an effective and safe method of administering analgesics, with a high degree of child and family satisfaction (Webb *et al*, 1989). However, individual child and family selection is important; PCA has been found to be useful in children as young as six years old (Berde *et al*, 1991).

The advantages of administering morphine in a PCA system as opposed to a continuous infusion include: increased user satisfaction (Webb *et al*, 1989), no delay between the perception of pain and administration of analgesia (Bray *et al*, 1996), greater user control (Carter, 1994), an overall reduction in analgesia used, with less sedation (Webb *et al*, 1989). A potential area of conflict with the use of PCA is that the number of attempts to administer analgesia versus the number of successes can vary between 35–94 percent (Rauen and Ho, 1989). The reasons for these discrepancies could include inappropriate infusion lock-out times, inadequate child education and inadequate assessment of child's individual needs. For PCA to be successful, staff must have adequate education (knowledge of pain management in children and be skilled in the use of equipment), and the child and family must have detailed preparation, including opportunity to become familiar with the equipment. Potential hazards of PCA include:

- Failure to load the pump correctly

- Failure to prepare the infusion correctly

- Failure in programming the pump

- Failure to check/regularly change disposable equipment for any faults (overuse can crack/break syringes or tubing)

- Failure to ensure environment is safe and prevent accidental drug administration

- Failure to prevent back siphoning of the drug into other infusions (if a designated cannula is not available) by not using a one-way anti-reflux and anti-syphon valve

- Overdose (could be due to prescribing error in both background infusion and bolus doses)
- Bolus given if drug line is flushed
- Failure to ensure cannula patency
- Equipment malfunction
- Poor, or errors in, documentation
- Inadequate training of staff
- Inadequate preparation and education of the child and family.

(Carter, 1994)

These can apply equally to continuous morphine infusions. *Appendix IV* outlines the key factors that should be considered when formulating local guidelines relating to the management and care of children with a morphine infusion (either continuous or via a PCA system).

Continuous infusions and PCA can also be administered subcutaneously. Doyle *et al*'s (1994) study suggests there are no differences in the effectiveness of intravenous compared with subcutaneous morphine using a PCA system. However, the subcutaneous route has several advantages; there may be less analgesia utilised (the subcutaneous uptake of morphine requires further research), reduced hypoxic episodes, and there is no need for a dedicated cannula (an important consideration for children with poor intravenous access) (Doyle *et al*, 1994). Despite these advantages, continuous subcutaneous morphine infusions do not appear to be widely used in clinical settings. In children maintaining the needle position may be problematic.

Epidural analgesia techniques are increasingly being used in the child health setting as the method of choice for relieving post-operative pain, particularly in thoracic and abdominal surgery. Epidural analgesia is thought to be more effective than other techniques, because significantly smaller drug doses can be used with profound analgesic effects (Chaney, 1995). Improved patient mobilisation (Brodner *et al*, 2001) results in better patient-outcomes and reduces hospital stay (Buggy and Smith,

1999). The technique involves the insertion of a fine-bore catheter, using a sterile procedure, into the epidural space at the level of the surgical incision, through which drugs can be administered either by a bolus injection or continuous infusion. The epidural space is the potential space between the dura mater (outer layer of the membranes which cover the brain and spinal cord) and the vertebral bones of the spine, and extends from the foramen magnum at the base of the skull to the sacral hiatus at the base of the spine. Nerve routes pass through this layer as they leave and enter the spinal canal; therefore, any drug given into the epidural space can have an effect directly on local nerves. In practice, a combination of drugs is often used to produce the desired effect: a local anaesthetic that blocks the transmission of nerve impulses within the spinal nerve root (sensory, motor and autonomic nerve fibres) and an opioid analgesia that acts on opioid receptors within the spinal cord. Some systemic absorption of the opioid drugs has the additional benefit of a sedative effect. Lejus *et al* (2001) found excellent analgesia was obtained in children with continuous epidural infusions using a combination of fentanyl (opioid) and bupivacaine (local anesthetic), with minimal side-effects. This combination seems to be commonly used in the paediatric setting. Fentanyl appears to be the opioid of choice because of its shorter onset of action and the ability to remain near the injection site, producing effective analgesia at the wound site. Its reduced duration of action results in the drug being cleared relatively quickly from the body once the infusion has been discontinued.

The side-effects of opioids given via an epidural will be similar to intravenous route, including pruritus, respiratory depression, nausea and vomiting, and urinary retention. However, the actual amount of drug used is much less and side-effects appear to be minimal in children (Lejus *et al*, 2001). Side-effects of local anaesthetic agents, including vasodilatation and hypotension, cardiotoxicity and central nervous system toxicity, have been reported in adult literature (Sasada and Smith, 1997). In addition, the procedure itself has potential complications, such as accidental puncture of the dura (with CSF loss), haematoma at the puncture site, misplacement of the catheter intrathecally (resulting in spinal anaesthesia), rostral spread of the drugs (if the nerve block reaches the level of the third, fourth or fifth cervical vertebrae, the diaphragm will become paralysed with respiratory failure) and infection (local abscess or meningitis). *Appendix IV* also outlines the key factors that should be considered when formulating local guidelines relating to the management and care of children with a continuous epidural infusion.

Non-pharmacological interventions

Non-pharmacological interventions for relieving pain should be used to support pharmacological interventions (Wood, 2002). There is no evidence to support their sole use in acute situations. The use of non-pharmacological interventions as adjunctive strategies, particularly in reducing the intensity of pain (Twycross, 1998b) and distress and anxiety of the child (May, 1992), should not be underestimated. Two studies (Unruh *et al*, 1983; Woodgate and Kristjanson, 1995), exploring children's perceptions of treating pain, clearly indicated that children manage and cope with pain through coping strategies, such as resting, applying pressure, patting, rubbing, sleeping and distraction (watching television, colouring, reading). Giving medication did not really feature in the child's view. Non-pharmacological interventions suitable for use in children include:

- Provision of appropriate information
- Play and activity therapy
- Distraction
- Application of heat and cold
- Non-nutritive sucking in neonates and infants
- Relaxation techniques
- Imagery
- Massage
- Therapeutic touch
- Aromatherapy

- Transcutaneous electrical nerve stimulation (TENS)
- Acupuncture
- Hypnosis.

(Carter, 1994; Eland, 1990; Twycross, 1998b)

Many of these techniques do not have a strong evidence base to support their effectiveness, and responses will be variable between children and across the age span. Some of these techniques may be more suitable in the management of chronic pain and may require specialist training.

There are relatively few studies that have examined if non-pharmacological interventions for relieving pain are used in clinical practice. Pölkki *et al*'s (2001) survey of nurses suggests non-pharmacological interventions, such as emotional support, providing preparatory information, distraction, helping with activities of daily living, maintaining a comfortable environment, positioning children, and touch, are frequently used. Other methods, such as TENS, were seldom used, with imagery, thermal regulation and massage only used occasionally. Lack of education and training in more complex non-pharmacological interventions may account for their limited use in clinical areas.

5.5 Improving pain management in children

Pain management needs to become imbedded into everyday practice, if it is to become effective for all children (Cummings *et al*, 1996). The *National Service Framework for Children, Standards for Hospital Services* (Department of Health, 2003) stresses the need for children to have appropriate prevention, assessment and control of their pain. This requires a radical change in working practices and attitudes towards children's pain management, education of the multi-disciplinary team, development of guidelines and protocols in relation to pain management, ongoing review and audit of practice and, most importantly, involving and supporting parents in the management of their child's pain.

Pain services

Acute post-operative pain should be managed by an acute pain team (Hogg, 1994; Lloyd-Thomas and Howard, 1994; Royal College of Anaesthetists, 2001; 2000; Royal College of Nursing, 1999; 1994; Royal College of Paediatrics and Child Health, 1997; Sanders and Michel, 2002). Within the UK, there has been a dramatic increase in the number of pain teams, with almost 88 percent of hospital trusts having a dedicated adult pain team (Clinical Standards Advisory Group, 2000). The Clinical Standards Advisory Group's research relating to the access and availability of pain services included children. However, the findings were disappointing, with only 50 percent of hospital trusts identified as having a pain service for children. This figure does not differentiate between designated paediatric pain teams and adult services providing an advisory service for children. It appears children are being disadvantaged. In addition to the disparity of service provision, there is no national consensus relating to the structure and function of pain teams (Sanders and Michel, 2002).

The UK Royal College of Paediatrics and Child Health (1997) suggests a pain service should consist of an interdisciplinary team, responsible for the development and implementation of guidelines and protocols relating to the management of pain in children. The structure of the service should consider the range of healthcare professionals necessary to provide the service (nurses, anaesthetists, surgeons, pharmacists, physiotherapists and psychologists) and their role within the team, the environment where the child is nursed and the availability of any specialised equipment (Lloyd-Thomas and Howard, 1994). The function of an acute pain team includes:

- Developing protocols for the assessment of pain

- Developing systems for including the child and family in the assessment process and subsequent management strategies

- Developing and providing child and parent information in a variety of formats

- Ensuring pain assessment tools which link to guidelines on analgesia choices (for example, a pain ladder)

- Developing and implementing care plans for complex analgesia interventions, such as continuous morphine infusions, PCA and epidural analgesia

- Developing guidelines on child observations, for example cardiovascular observations, pain assessment and sedation scores, and the frequency of recordings

- Developing an overall management strategy (such as an acute pain management algorithm) (*Figure 5.4c*).

(Royal College of Anaesthetists, 2001; 2000)

One of the functions of an acute pain team must be ongoing audit, which enables standards to be monitored and should be linked to future developments and identify potential research areas (Goddard and Pickup, 1996; Lloyd-Thomas and Howard, 1994; Sherwood, 1998). Routine data should be collected in relation to:

- The number of children who have had pain scores recorded post-operatively

- The number of children with unacceptable pain scores post-operatively

- The number of children visited by a member of the acute pain team post-operatively

- The number of children with advanced analgesia techniques (continuous morphine infusions, PCA, epidural infusions)

- The number of children who have had a daily visit from a member of the acute pain team.

(Royal College of Anaesthetists, 2001; 2000)

If the quality of care is to be improved, the data collected should be regularly reviewed, where current practice can be compared with the standards set and an action plan to remedy any deficiencies (Crombie *et al*, 1993).

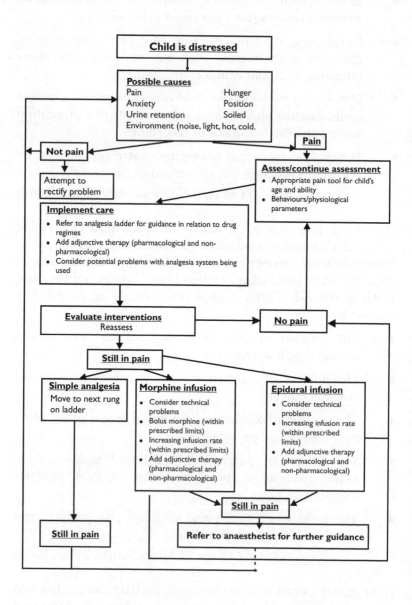

Figure 5.4c: Example of an acute post-operative pain management algorithm

Although having an effective pain team is important, improving pain management does not have to be a complex process and much can be achieved if every healthcare professional caring for children adhere to principles of good practice, including:

- Communicating effectively with children and asking them how they feel and how much pain they have

- Listening to children and understanding their fears and anxieties, such as avoiding the use of injections

- Observing children and recognising both physiological and behavioural indicators of pain

- Ensuring effective education of the child and family (both verbal and written) in relation to pain, and offering realistic choices

- Involving children in choice of assessment tool

- Ensuring a range of pain management strategies is available

- Ensuring clear and concise documentation, evaluating the effectiveness of treatments

- Involving the family in care and respecting their wishes.

Training and education

There is a need for effective training and education in relation to children's pain management, for all healthcare professionals. From a nursing perspective, this should begin with a re-evaluation of the content of pre-registration courses in relation to the theoretical input relating to children's pain (Twycross, 2001). The limited time devoted to pain management in educational curricula may subconsciously be influencing the lack of priority pain management has in practice. The lack of accredited education opportunities available in the management of children's pain places increased importance on formal education in the clinical setting. Education packages can influence the implementation of pain assessment tools and change opinions about pain management in children (Twycross, 1997). Understanding pain in children increases concurrently with the academic qualifications of nurses, which influences clinical decision-making (Margolius *et al*, 1995).

Education is vital if the implementation of guidelines and policies is to be successful (Effective Health Care Bulletin, 1994). For change to occur, active dissemination strategies are essential (Thomas *et al*, 1999), including educational packages, raising the profile of pain at ward and unit levels, and having a visible member of the pain team available to support ward staff and troubleshoot potential problems. This is not possible without a dedicated team of staff.

Family-centred care and pain management

It is essential that healthcare professionals involve parents in the process of managing their child's pain because:

- Parents are an invaluable source of information about a child's normal behaviours and can assist in the assessment of pain, particularly in relation to non-verbal cues

- Parents have intimate knowledge of a child's usual coping mechanisms

- The presence of parents greatly reduces the anxiety provoked by hospitalisation

- Parents will know the child's normal comforters

- Involving parents in managing pain is essential in cases where early discharge from hospital necessitates that pain management continues at home.

(Twycross, 1998)

Unfortunately, recent studies by Byrne *et al* (2001), Simons *et al* (2001,) and Pölkki *et al* (2002) suggest that, in reality, parental involvement in pain management occurs at very superficial levels, with parents having very passive roles in the overall management of their child's pain. Again it appears nurses need to be much better educated in all aspects of pain management in children and realise that this lack of knowledge is hindering children's nurses in their ability to support parents. Including parents in their child's pain management can be achieved by:

- Introducing issues relating to pain management and potential roles for parents during the admission procedure

- Providing written information relating to pain management

- Providing parents with guidance in relation to non-pharmacological methods of pain management

- Ensuring emotional support is provided in order to prevent parents from feeling isolated and helpless.

(Byrne et al, 2001; Pölkki et al, 2002; Simons et al, 2001)

Many of the key principles enshrined within the concept of family-centred care (Nethercott, 1993: section 2.1) are particularly pertinent to managing pain in children and include:

- Understanding the family's social, cultural and religious context

- Valuing parents' contribution to the overall management of their child's pain

- Providing explicit information to enable parents to participate in decision-making and the acquisition of knowledge pertaining to their child's illness

- Involving the prime care-giver in the pain assessment process and evaluating the effectiveness of strategies

- Involving families in technical aspects of care, in accordance with their own perceived abilities and willingness to develop the necessary skills

- Continuing usual child care/comforting practices

- Providing parents with support and encouragement in order to reduce stress and anxiety

- Evaluating the impact of the sick child on the family and taking steps to ensure support continues as needed after discharge, or in the event of death.

If these principles are applied, there is potential to improve the pain management of children. Assessing pain in children, and in particular children with profound special needs, is a challenge (Carter *et al*, 2002a). Unfortunately, the drive towards shorter hospital stays and the shifting of care to the primary health setting has generally not been reflected in an increase in primary care service provision (Bridger and Rees, 1995). Parents inevitably take on the responsibility for ongoing care of the child following discharge (Ireland and Rushforth, 1998). This is an onerous responsibility and can be a daunting prospect for many families and children, and will include the need to manage the child's pain. Prior to discharge, the child and family will require detailed advice in relation to pain management, including explanations of take-home analgesia, and education relating to non-pharmacological strategies that may alleviate the child's pain (Päivi K *et al*, 2003). Therefore, it is vital that nurses understand the wider concepts of pain management. Children's nurses must ensure parents are educated and supported when taking on the responsibility of managing their child's pain.

References

Baker C, Wong D (1987) QUESTT; a process of pain assessment in nursing. *Orthopaedic Nurs* 6(1): 11–21

Berde CB, Sethna NF (2002) Drug therapy: analgesics for the treatment of pain in children. *N Engl J Med* 347(14): 1094–103

Berde CB, Lehn BM, Yee JD *et al* (1991) Patient-controlled analgesia in children and adolescents: a randomized, prospective comparison with intramuscular administration of morphine for postoperative analgesia. *J Pediatrics* 118: 460–66

Bieri D, Reeve RA, Champion GD *et al* (1990) The faces pain scale for the self assessment of the severity of pain experienced by children: development, initial validation and preliminary investigation for ratio scale properties. *Pain* 41: 139–50

Bray RJ (1983) Post-operative analgesia provided by morphine infusion in children. *Anaesthesia* 38: 1075–78

Bray RJ, Woodhams AM, Vallis CJ *et al* (1996) A double-blind comparison of morphine infusion and patient controlled analgesia in children. *Paediatr Anaesthesiol* 6: 121–27

Bray RJ, Beeton MB, Hinton W, Seviour JA (1986) Plasma morphine levels produced by continuous infusion in children. *Anaesthesia* **41**: 753–55

Bridger P, Rees M (1995) What a difference a day makes. *Health Services J* **105**: 22–23

Broadbent C (2000) The pharmacology of acute pain. *Nurs Times* **96**(26): 39–41

Brodner G, Van Aken H, Hertle L *et al* (2001) Multimodal perioperative management-combined thoracic epidural analgesia, forced mobilization, and oral nutrition reduces hormonal stress and improves convalescence after major urologic surgery. *Anesthesia Analgesia* **92**(60): 1594–600

Buckingham S (1993) Pain scales for toddlers *Nurs Stand* **7**(25Supp): 12–13

Buggy DJ, Smith G (1999) Epidural anaesthesia and analgesia: better outcome after major surgery? Growing evidence suggests so. *Br Med J* **319**(7209): 530–31

Burr S (1993) Myths in practice. *Nurs Stand* **7**(25Suppl): 4–5

Byrne A, Morton J, Salmon P (2001) Defending against patients' pain. A qualitative analysis of nurses' responses to children's postoperative pain. *J Psychosom Res* **50**: 69–76

Carr ECJ (1997) Evaluating the use of a pain assessment tool and care plan: a pilot study. *J Adv Nurs* **26**: 1073–79

Carter B (1994) *Child and Infant Pain: Principles of Nursing Care and Management*. Chapman and Hall, London

Carter B, Lambrenos K, Thursfield J (2002) A pain workshop: an approach to eliciting the views of young people with chronic pain. *J Clin Nurs* **11**(6): 753–62

Carter B, McArthur E, Cunliffe M (2002a) Dealing with uncertainty: parental assessment of pain in their children with profound special needs. *J Adv Nurs* **38**(5): 449–57

Chaney MA (1995) Side effects of intrathecal and epidural opiods. *Can J Anesthesia* **42**(10): 891–903

Clinical Standards Advisory Group (2000) *Services for Patients with Pain*. Stationery Office, London

Crombie I K, Davies HTO, Abraham CSC, Florey C duc V (1993) *The Audit Handbook; Improving Health Care Through Clinical Audit*. John Wiley and Sons, Chichester

Cummings EA, Reid GJ, Finley A *et al* (1996) Prevalence and source of pain management in pediatric inpatients. *Pain* **68**: 25–31

Department of Health (2003) *Getting the Right Start: National Service Framework for Children. Standards for Hospital Services.* Stationery Office, London

Doyle E, Morton NS, McNicol (1994) Comparison of patient-controlled analgesia in children by i.v. and s.c. routes of administration. *Br J Anaesthesia* 72: 533–36

Effective Health Care Bulletin (1994) *Implementing Clinical Guidelines.* 8, NHS Centre for Reviews and Dissemination, University of York

Eland J (1990) Pain in children. *Nurs Clin N Am* 24(40): 871–74

Eland J (1981) Minimizing pain associated with prekindergarten intramuscular injections. *Iss Comprehen Pediatr Nurs* 5: 361–72

Eland J, Anderson M (1977) The experience of pain in children. In: Jacox AK, ed. *Pain: A Source Book for Nurses and Other Health Care Professionals.* Little, Brown and Company, Boston

Fitzgerald M, Beggs S (2001) The neurobiology of pain: developmental aspects. *Neuroscientist* 7: 246–57

Fitzgerald M, Koltzenberg M (1986) The functional development of inhibitory pathways in the dorsolateral finiculus of the newborn rat spinal cord. *Brain Res* 389: 261–70

Gaffney A, McGrath PJ, Dick B (2003) Measuring pain in children: developmental and instrument issues. In: Schechter NL, Berde CB, Yester M, eds. *Pain in Infants, Children and Adolescents*, 2nd edn. Lippincott, Williams and Wilkins, Philadelphia

Goddard JM, Pickup SE (1996) Postoperative pain in children. Combining audit and a clinical nurse specialist to improve management. *Anaesthesia* 51: 533–36

Hawley DD (1984) Post-operative pain in children: misconceptions, descriptions and interventions. *Pediatr Nurs* 10: 20–23

Hawthorn J, Redmond K (1998) *Pain Causes and Management.* Blackwell Science, Oxford

Heuther SE, Leo J (2002) Pain, temperature regulation, sleep and sensory function. In: McCance KL, Huether SE, eds. *Pathophysiology: The Biological Basis for Disease in Adults and Children*, 4th edn. Mosby, St Louis

Hogg C (1994) *Setting Standards for Children Undergoing Surgery.* Action for Sick Children, London

Hurley A, Whelan EG (1988) Cognitive development and children's perception of pain. *Pediatr Nurs* 14(1): 21– 24

International Association for the Study of Pain (1992). *Management of Acute Pain: A Practical Guide.* IASP Press, Seattle

Ireland L, Rushforth H (1998) Day care—in whose best interests? *Paediatr Nurs* **10**(5): 15–19

Jackson KL (1995) The state we're in. *Child Health* **3**(1): 14–17

Jacob E, Puntillo KA (1999) A survey of nursing practice in the assessment and management of pain in children. *Pediatr Nurs* **25**(3): 278–86

La Fleur CJ, Raway B (1999) School-age child and adolescent perception of pain intensity. *Pediatr Nurs* **25**(1): 45–50; 55

Lejus C, Surbled M, Schowoerer D *et al* (2001) Postoperative epidural analgesia with bupivacaine and fentanly: hourly pain assessment in 348 paediatric cases. *Paediatr Anaesthesia* **11**(3): 327–32

Lloyd-Thomas AR, Howard RF (1994) A pain service for children. *Paediatr Anaesthesia* **4**: 3–15

Longstaff A (2000) *Instant Notes—Neuroscience*. BIOS Scientific Publications Ltd, Oxford

McCaffery M (1968) *Nursing Practice Theories Relating to cognition, bodily pain, and Man-Environment Interactions*. Lippincott, Los Angeles

Mackintosh C, Bowles S (2000) The effect of an acute pain service on nurses' knowledge and beliefs about post-operative pain. *J Clin Nurs* **9**(1): 119–26

McIlvaine WB (1989) Perioperative pain management in children: a review. *J Pain Sym Man* **4**(4): 215–29

Maikler VE (1998) Pharmacological pain management in children: a review of intervention research. *J Pediatr Nurs* **13**(1): 3–14

Margolius FR, Hudson KA, Michel Y (1995) Beliefs and perceptions about children in pain; a survey. *Pediatr Nurs* **21**(2): 111–15; 132–33

Mather L, Mackie J (1983) The incidence of post-operative pain in children. *Pain* **15**: 271–82

May L (1992) Reducing pain and anxiety in children. *Nurs Stand* **6**(4): 25–28

Moriarty A (1998) The pharmacological management of acute pain. In: Twycross A, Moriarty A, Betts T, eds. *Paediatric Pain Management: a Multidisciplinary Approach*. Radcliffe, Oxford

National Prescribing Center (2000) The use of oral analgesics in primary care. *MeReC Bull* **11**(1): 1–4

Nethercott S (1993) A concept for all the family, family centred care: a concept analysis. *Profess Nurse* **8**(12): 794–97

Newell P (1991) *The United Nations Convention and Children's Rights in the UK*. National Children's Bureau, London

Nursing and Midwifery Council (2002) *The Code of Professional Conduct.* NMC, London

Piaget J (1952) *The Origins of Intelligence in Children.* International Universities Press, New York

Päivi K, Vehviläinen-Julkunen K, Pietilä AM *et al* (2003) Parents' use of nonpharmacological methods to alleviate children's postoperative pain at home. *J Adv Nurs* **41**(4): 367–75

Pölkki T, Vehviläinen-Julkunen K, Pietilä AM *et al* (2002) Parental views on participation in their child's pain relief measures and recommendations to healthcare providers. *J Pediatr Nurs* **17**(4): 270–77

Pölkki T, Vehviläinen-Julkunen K, Pietilä AM (2001) Nonpharmacological methods in relieving children's postoperative pain: a survey on hospital nurses in Finland. *J Adv Nurs* **34**(4): 483–92

Rauen KH, Ho M (1989) Children's use of patient controlled analgesia in pediatric surgery. *Pediatr Nurs* **15**(6): 589–93.

Royal College of Anaesthetists (2001) *Guidance on the Provision of Paediatric Anaesthetic Services.* RCA, London

Royal College of Anaesthetists (2000) *Raising the Standard.* RCA, London

Royal College of Nursing (1999) *Clinical practice guidelines: the recognition and assessment of acute pain in children.* RCN, London

Royal College of Nursing (1994) *Standards of Care in Paediatric Nursing,* 2nd edn. RCN, Harrow

Royal College of Paediatrics and Child Health (1997) *Prevention and Control of Pain in Children—A Manual for Health Care Professionals.* BMJ Publishing, London

Sanders MK, Michel MZM (2002) Acute pain services—how effective are we? *Anaesthesia* **57**(9): 927–28

Sasada M, Smith S (1997) *Drugs in Anaesthesia and Intensive Care.* Oxford Medical Publications, Oxford

Schechter NL, Allen DA, Hanson K (1986) Status of pediatric pain control: a comparison of hospital analgesic usage in children and adults. *Pediatrics* **77**(1): 11–15

Schofield P (1995) Using pain assessment tools to help patents. *Profess Nurse* **10**(11): 703–706

Sherwood P (1998) Auditing paediatric pain management. *Paediatr Pain* **10**(6): 15–17

Simons J, Franck L, Roberson E (2001) Parent involvement in children's pain care: views of parents and nurses. *J Adv Nurs* **36**(4): 591–99

Stevens B, Koren G (1998) Evidence-based pain management for infants. *Curr Opin Pediatr* **10**(2): 203–207

Tatman A, Johnson P (1998) Pain assessment in the pre-verbal child. In: Twycross A, Moriarty A, Betts T, eds. *Paediatric Pain Management: A Multidisciplinary Approach*. Radcliffe, Oxon

Taylor A (1998) Pain assessment in children. In: Twycross A, Moriarty A, Betts T, eds. *Paediatric Pain Management: A Multidisciplinary Approach*. Radcliffe, Oxon

Thomas L H, McColl E, Cullum N, *et al* (1999) Clinical guidelines in nursing, midwifery and the therapies: a systematic review. *J Adv Nurs* **30**(1): 40–50

Thompson KL, Varni JW (1986) A developmental cognitive-biobehavioral approach to pediatric pain assessment. *Pain* **25**: 283–66

Twycross A (2002) Managing pain in children: an observational study. *NT Res* **7**(3): 164–78

Twycross A (2002a) Educating nurses about pain management: the way forward. *J Clin Nurs* **11**(6): 705–14

Twycross A (2001) Achieving consensus about pain content for child branch curricula. *J Adv Nurs* **34**(1): 51–60

Twycross A (1998) Perceptions about paediatric pain. In: Twycross A, Moriarty A, Betts T, eds. *Paediatric Pain Management: A Multidisciplinary Approach*. Radcliffe, Oxon

Twycross A (1998a) Children's cognitive level and their perception of pain. *Paediatr Nurs* **10**(3): 24–27

Twycross A (1998b) Non-drug methods of pain control. In: Twycross A, Moriarty A, Betts T, eds. *Paediatric Pain Management: A Multidisciplinary Approach*. Radcliffe, Oxon

Twycross A (1997) Nurses' perceptions of pain in children. *Paediatr Nurs* **9**(1): 16–9.

Twycross A, Mayfield C, Savory J (1999) Pain management for children with special needs: a neglected area? *Paediatr Nurs* **11**(6): 43–45

Unruh A, McGrath P, Cunningham SJ, Humphreys P (1983) Children's drawings of their pain. *Pain* **17**: 385–92.

Volpe J (1981) *Neurology of the Newborn*. Saunders Philadelphia.

Walco GA, Cassidy RC, Schechter NL (1994) Pain, hurt and harm: the ethics of pain control in infants and children. *N Engl J Med* **331**(8): 541–44

Wall PD, Melzack R (1989) *Textbook of Pain*. Churchill Livingstone, London

Children's surgical nursing: principles and practice

Webb CJ, Stergios DA, Rogers BM (1989) Patient-controlled analgesics as postoperative pain treatment for children. *J Pediatr Nurs* **4**(3): 126–71

Wills L (2002) Managing change through audit: post-operative pain in ambulatory care. *Paediatr Nurs* **14**(9): 35–38

Wood S (2002) Pain: assessment and diagnosis. *Nurs Times* **98**(39): 43–46

Wood S (2002a) Pain: Nursing care and implications for nursing. *Nurs Times* **98**(40): 39–42

Woodgate R, Kristjanson LJ (1995) Young children's behavioural responses to acute pain: strategies for getting better. *J Adv Nurs* **22**(2): 243–49

Wong D, Baker C (1988) Pain in children: comparison of assessment scales. *Pediatr Nurs* **14**(1): 9–17

World Health Organization (1998) Cancer Pain Relief and Palliative Care in Children. World Health Organization, Geneva

Yaster M, Deshpande JK (1988) Management of pediatric pain with opioid analgesics. *Pediatrics* **113**: 421–29

SIX

WOUND CARE

Greater understanding of the physiological processes of wound healing, technological advances and the increasingly complex nature of wounds, has resulted in wound care becoming a specialism within its own right (Baxter, 2001). Although specialist practitioners and consultant nurses have vital roles to play in terms of developing and advancing wound care through education, promoting evidence-based practice, providing expert advice, consultancy and liaison roles, undertaking advanced interventions, developing guidelines and monitoring quality (Gibson and Bamford, 2001; Harker, 2001), it is essential for all nurses caring for patients with wounds to understand and apply the principles of wound care to their client group. Annually, 1.3 million children are treated for minor injuries (cuts, lacerations), and 500,000 children undergo surgical operations (House of Commons Health Select Committee, 1997), resulting in wounds being common in children. Most of these are quick to heal and do not require complex care (Casey, 2001). However, all wounds require appropriate management in terms of the correct type of cleansing, dressing, promoting factors which encouraging healing, and providing the child and family with appropriate education, support and guidance.

This chapter will outline the care and management of a child and family where the child has a surgical wound. Section one describes the different types of wounds and the process of wound healing, which must be understood in order to recognising normal/abnormal tissue responses and provide effective wound care (Dealey, 1999). The second section will focus upon practical issues relating to managing surgical wounds, and the recognition and management of complications.

6.1 Classification of wounds and the physiology of wound healing

Classification of wounds

The labelling of wounds varies and can be related to:

1. *Acute/chronic/post-operative* (Dealey, 1999)

   a. Acute wounds: are traumatic wounds as a result of an accident

   b. Post-operative wounds: are intentional acute wounds

   c. Chronic wounds: can be either wounds that are difficult to heal or classified as chronic due to the underlying cause such as vascular disorders.

2. *Type of wound closure*

   Surgical wounds are often described in terms of how the wound site is closed. Moore and Foster (2002) described three main types of wound closures:

   a. *Primary closure*—sometimes referred to as healing by primary or first intention: the deep structures and wound edges are brought together in close opposition. The aim is to bring the tissues together in anatomical layers without tension, which are then secured, for example, with sutures

   b. *Primary closure with insertion of a drain*: if the tissues can be brought together, but there is a cavity, or potential cavity, due to possible buildup of pus, fluid or blood within the wound, the insertion of a drain will be necessary

   c. *Open wounds or healing by secondary intention*: it may not always be possible to perform a primary closure, for example, in infected wounds or where there has been extensive tissue loss. The wound can either be left open to heal naturally or be closed at a later date (delayed primary closure); the choice will depend upon the underlying reason for leaving the wound open and the predicted rate of the healing process.

3. *Depth of the wound* (Dealey, 1999):

   a. Partial thickness wounds: the skins dermal layer, hair follicle shafts and sweat glands remain intact
   b. Full thickness wounds: the dermis is destroyed and there is destruction of deeper tissues.

4. *Wound appearance* (Dealey, 1999):

   a. *Epithelialising tissue*: new epithelial tissue has a pinky-white colour, the wound margins become slightly raised as the epithelial cells initially divide, but the wound flattens as the cells migrate across the wound. In large wounds, there will be patches of epithelial cells on the wound surface
   b. *Granulation tissue*: the wound is red and appears globular due to presence of capillary loops. The vascular state of the wound makes it prone to bleeding
   c. *Sloughy wounds*: there is a white/yellow exudates on the wound surface made up of dead cells and this is a normal part of the inflammatory process
   d. *Infected wounds*: the wound will have increased redness at the wound margins, discolouration of wound bed, increased exudates production, increased pain and heat, and there may be an offensive smell
   e. *Necrotic wounds*: the wound appears brown/black and is a result of cellular death due to ischaemia. Removal of the necrotic area is necessary for the wound to heal.

The process of wound healing

The natural physiological processes that occur in wound healing are highly complex. For convenience, wound healing is usually described in stages; these stages overlap and the process is continuous. Unfortunately, the description of these stages varies:

- Inflammation, granulation and maturation (Casey, 1998)
- Inflammation, reconstruction, epithelialisation, and maturation (Dealey, 1999)
- Inflammation, granulation, epithelialisation, and remodelling (Moore and Foster, 2002; Russell, 2002)

- Inflammatory, destructive, proliferative and maturation (Shipperley and Martin, 2002).

However, the actual chemical and biological reactions that occur, despite labelling differences, are described consistently. Inflammation, granulation, epithelialisation, and remodelling (Moore and Foster, 2002; Russell, 2002) will be outlined (*Table 6.1a*), because the terminology of the stages appears to represent the actual cellular processes occurring. Depending upon the type of wound and stage of the healing, a combination of healing stages can be visualised together in some wounds. The vast majority of surgical wounds heal by first intention (Gould, 2001). *Table 6.1a* describes the stages of wound healing for primary closed wounds.

Factors that affect wound healing

1. Age

Age has been identified as an important factor with the potential to affect wound healing (Dealey, 1999). Certainly studies relating to wound healing in the elderly population (reviewed in Morison *et al*, 1997) indicate that there is decreased efficiency in wound healing with age, particularly over 85 years of age. Morrison *et al* indicate that the faster wound healing rate in children could be due to normal physiological changes in the dermis of the skin. The dermis increases in thickness during the first years of life, doubling in thickness by seven years of age. This increased activity has the potential to assist wound healing in children. In addition, children will not have the systematic diseases associated with adults, in particular cardiovascular disease and complications of diabetes, which may compromise circulation and therefore tissue perfusion.

Table 6.1a: Stages of wound healing, appearance and healing by primary intention

Stage of wound healing (Adapted from Moore and Foster, 2002; Russell, 2002)	Appearance (Adapted from Dealey, 1999)	Healing by primary intention (Adapted from Heath, 1998)
Inflammation Following tissue damage, a series of reactions occurs: Initially, blood vessels constrict in an attempt to reduce blood loss, and the clotting process is initiated (platelet aggregation and formation of a fibrin mesh) in order to seal the damaged surface. Within about an hour following injury, reactions within the clotting process lead to the release of chemicals, such as histamine, prostaglandin and serotonin, resulting in vasodilation, increased capillary permeability, attracting white blood cells and release of growth factors into the injury site. The first white cells to arrive are the neutrophils whose phagocytic action removes toxins and dead cells. Increased blood supply is essential to bring white cells, oxygen and nutrients to the site. When active, neutrophils have a relatively short lifespan. Macrophages enter the site at about two days, and continue to remove cellular debris, worn out neutrophils and any bacteria entering the wound, and release specific growth factors. The inflammatory phase lasts about 3–5 days.	**Inflammation** The four cardinal signs which occur as a result of the inflammatory process are: *Redness* as a result of vasodilation and increased blood flow. *Heat* as a result of increased metabolic activity. *Swelling* as a result of vasodilation and increased permeability of capillaries, allowing cells and fluid to pass into the wound site. *Pain* can be a result of physical or chemical damage to nerve endings, or from pressure due to swelling. The activity of the neutrophils in removing debris from the wound gives it a characteristic 'yellow' appearance. Infection or presence of foreign material will prolong the inflammatory phase.	Immediately after the surgical incision, temporary vasoconstriction reduces blood supply. This is quickly followed by the inflammatory response. Epidermis Dermis Subcutaneous tissue The wound margins are held together, for example by sutures, fluid fills the space between the wound margins, healing by primary intention can begin.

Stage of wound healing (Adapted from Moore and Foster, 2002; Russell, 2002)	Appearance (Adapted from Dealey, 1999)	Healing by primary intention (Adapted from Heath, 1998)
Granulation There is active regeneration of new tissue, such as capillaries, collagen and connective tissue, under the influence of the biochemical activity of the macrophages, endothelial cells and platelets. Initially, it is the fibroblasts that form the scaffolding for the collagen proteins, which give strength to the wound. As the granulation tissue is formed, the wound begins to contract with approximation of the edges of the wound. The length of this stage varies considerably depending upon the size of the wound from 4–5 days in primary closure and up to 24 days in large open wounds.	**Granulation** This stage will not really be visible in wounds that have been primary closed. In open wounds, the area will appear red and vascular. The surface is very fragile with the capillary vessels easily disrupted (bleeds easily).	8 hours post surgery: a blood clot fills the wound, the area becomes walled off, neutrophils begin to phagocytise cell debris. 16 hours onwards: there is epithelialisation of the surface of the wound. 24–48 hours post surgery: cells below the epithelial layer begin to unite; however, the wound has poor tensile strength
Epithelialisation Growth factors stimulate proliferation and migration of squamous epithelial cells from the margin of the wound. This stage can only progress if the tissue underneath is viable and the environment is moist. When cells meet in the centre of the wound, contact inhibition prevents excessive proliferation of epithelial cells. The length of this stage is variable.	**Epithelialisation** The wound is a pink-white colour with a translucent appearance. If the wound is extensive, there may be patches of epithelial cells on top of an expanse of granulation tissue.	Between 5–12 days there is maximum increase in tensile strength. Sutures can be removed, the actual timing will depend upon assessment of the wound, tissue healing, depth of wound and area of the body. Scar tissue slowly increases in strength and by one month is 70–80% of the original skin strength.
Remodelling The newly formed granulation tissue and epithelial cells require remodelling to become comparable to normal tissue structures and function properly. The vascularisation initially required is no longer necessary and the random pattern of the collagen fibres becomes more structured, adding strength to the wound. If a scab has formed, this will detach and leave new tissue underneath. The scar gradually flattens. The process can continue from one month to a year.	**Remodelling** Eventually the scar will be smooth, and have a white appearance.	The eventual white scar is the result of deposition and contraction of collagen in the wound and thickening of the skin over the wound.

2. Wound environment

Active cells within the wound require an optimal environment to maintain effective functioning (Casey, 1999). Cells function best at body temperature and in high humidity, therefore a warm and moist environment will encourage wound healing. Even though the evidence supporting moist wound healing has been available since the 1960s, implementation has been slow (Baxter, 2002). Although a moist wound promotes healing, excessive moisture or bathing in large amounts of fluid delays healing by causing maceration of the granulation tissue and surrounding skin (Casey, 1999). Swabbing wounds with gauze and cotton wool, for example to clean a wound, will damage the surface of the wound and delay healing (Parker, 2000; Towler, 2001).

3. Presence of infection

The presence of infection delays wound healing. Systemic infection reduces the availability of white cells for wound healing (Dealey, 1999). Infection in the actual wound prolongs the inflammatory stage of healing and therefore compromises the healing process (Dealey, 1999). In addition, the toxins produced by many bacteria impair normal cell function (White *et al*, 2002). Infection may cause dehiscence in a wound that has been primary closed. Infection is a major complication of hospital admissions, with an estimated 9 percent of all inpatients developing an infection (Emmerson *et al*, 1996). The rate of infection for clean surgical wounds has been estimated to be as high as 8 percent (Plowman *et al*, 1999; Reilly *et al*, 2001). Early studies focusing solely on children's wounds suggested surgical infection rates range from 2.5 percent to 20 percent (Doig and Wilkinson, 1976). More recently, Horwitz *et al*'s (1998) study of 846 children, who had undergone a range of procedures, demonstrated an overall wound infection of 4.4 percent. Although a much lower figure when compared with studies which contain both children and adults, it is still a significant number of children.

The main source of post-operative wound contamination appears to be during the actual surgical procedure (Horwitz *et al*, 1998). Intra-operative factors that increase the potential risk of developing a wound infection include the duration of the operation, skin preparation and type of suture material (Briggs, 1997). Minimising the risk of bacterial contamination in the theatre environment is an imperative part of intra-operative care (*Chapter 4*). The type of surgery influences the potential for post-operative wound infections. Surgery involving the gastro-intestinal tract, where there is a normal complement of bacteria, increases the risk of post-operative infection by 27 per-cent (Nichols, 1998). Therefore, prophylactic antibiotics for lengthy procedures and high infection risk surgery may be advis-able (Horwitz *et al*, 1998; Nichols, 1998). The physical status of the child does not appear to influence infection rates (Horwitz *et al*, 1998). However, many routine practices undertaken to pre-pare patients for theatre may contribute to the post-operative infections, both positively and negatively. These include bath-ing/showering and hair removal prior to surgery (Briggs, 1997) and are discussed in relation to peri-operative care in *Chapter 4*.

4. *Nutrition and drugs*

The physiological processes of wound healing are energy-dependent, and require a range of nutrients to sustain cellular actively (Dealey, 1999). Wound healing is dependent upon:

- Carbohydrates to maintain cellular activity, such as the metabolism of leucocytes and fibroblasts

- Proteins for the synthesis of inflammatory mediators and the development of granulation tissue, primarily the syn-thesis of collagen. In addition, in chronic wounds with heavy exudates, proteins can be lost in the exudates

- Vitamins (particularly A, B, C, K) and minerals (such as copper, iron, zinc), which are co-factors in many meta-bolic activities including those necessary in wound healing

- Fats for healthy synthesis of new cells.

(Gray and Cooper, 2001)

Inadequate nutrition may be a contributing factor in poor wound healing and the development of wound infections (Gray and Cooper, 2001). A nutritional assessment and ensuring an adequate dietary intake are essential if wound healing is to be promoted.

Drugs that affect normal cells division, suppress the inflammatory process or hinder the uptake of vitamins, for example immuno-suppressants and anti-inflammatory drugs have the potential to affect or delay wound healing. There may be a need for additional dietary supplements in children at risk of poor wound healing (Gray and Cooper, 2001).

5.   *Choice of wound dressing*

The purposes of a wound dressing are to provide protection and maintain an ideal wound healing environment (Casey, 1999). In addition to these passive functions, certain dressings can actively promote cellular activity and encourage healing (Lait and Smith, 1998). Delay in healing can be a result of poor choice of dressing. Unfortunately, nurses continue to use inappropriate dressings, due to an inability to keep abreast of new products, lack of education in wound healing and reliance on products they are familiar with (Lait and Smith, 1998). The ideal wound dressing should:

- Maintain high humidity
- Provide thermal insulation
- Remove excessive exudate
- Be impermeable to pathogens
- Allow trauma- and pain-free removal
- Not leave particles from the dressing in the wound
- Be cost effective
- Be easy to use
- Be comfortable and allow mobility
- Permit bathing
- Minimise the risk of cross-infection
- Be hypoallergenic.

(Casey, 1999; Watret and White, 2001)

In addition there should be consideration of:

● The child's stage of development (particularly if accidental removal is to be minimised in the young child)

● The preferences of the child and family

● The frequency of changes.

These latter aspects are particularly important if parents are expected to continue wound care and dressing changes, following discharge. Although there is no universal dressing, these factors, plus an assessment of the stage of healing and the type and position of the wound, should be considered when choosing a dressing. Despite the vast number of dressings now available, the majority fall into six main groups. *Table 6.1b* provides a summary of the main types of dressings and their main uses. The manufacturers' information should always be checked, which should provide information about the composition of the dressing, types of wound it may be applicable for use with, instructions for use and recommended times for changing the dressings. Furthermore, the dressing package should be checked to ensure the packaging is intact and the shelf life has not expired.

Table 6.1b: Types of dressings and their application (adapted from Casey, 2001; Russell, 2002)

Type of dressing product	Characteristic and main use
Woven dressings: dry gauze, paraffin impregnated gauze e.g. Jelonet® Paratulle® low adherent dressings e.g. Melolin® Release®	Generally inappropriate for primary contact with the wound because cells can migrate onto the surface of the dressing, often adhere to the wound, cause trauma to healing tissue on removal and do not promote moist wound environment. Usually used as absorbent medium for secondary dressing. (Silicon coated woven dressings, for example Mepitel®, can be used in direct contact with the wound.)
Film dressings e.g. Opsite® Tegaderm®	Permeable to water vapour and oxygen, impermeable to water and micro-organisms. Ensures a moist environment, convenient, allows observation of the wound. Suitable for wounds that have been primary closed and where there is not expected to be an exudate. They do not provide any insulation. Can be used as a secondary dressing to provide a waterproof surface.

Type of dressing product	Characteristic and main use
Hydrocolloids e.g. Granuflex® Comfeel ®	Manufactured from cellulose which is highly absorbent and when wet forms a gel which maintains a moist (but not wet) surface. Aids wound healing by a gentle debriding action. Impermeable to water and bacteria. Comes in many forms, such as wafers, gels, and powders or in a combination with other dressings. Absorbency between products varies. Selection and correct application of product important.
Hydrogels e.g. GranuGel ® Intrasite®	Composed of gel, which when in contact with a wound releases water. Main use is to rehydrate wounds, debride and clean sloughy or necrotic wounds. Painless to apply and remove, can be soothing. Not suitable if there is excessive exudate, and will be ineffective if used with highly absorbent dressings, such as hydrocolloids. Can causes maceration of healthy tissues around the wound if this is not protected.
Alginate e.g. Kaltostat® Sorbsan®	Composed of calcium alginate, extracted from seaweed, which is integrated into a woven dressing. When the dressing comes in contact with a wet environment, a gel is produced which acts as a gentle debrider. Depending upon type of alginate, once activated may stay as a gel (requiring irrigation to remove) or may form a compact dressing which can be removed in one piece. Alginates require sufficient exudate to be activated. Cannot be used on dry wounds.
Foams e.g. Allevn® Lyofoam®	Foam dressings are thick spongy dressings that can be moulded into difficult shaped wounds or around small body parts. They are designed to absorb large amounts of exudate, therefore cannot be used on low exudate wounds. They provide thermal insulation, do not shed particles, are non-adherent and easily removed.

6.2   The management of surgical wounds

Surgical wounds by their very nature are intentional; therefore theoretically, the potential risk of complications should be minimal. Management depends upon the type of wound, position of the wound and the needs of the child and family. The principles of managing wounds that have been primary closed, primary closed with insertion of a drain, and more complex surgical wounds will be outlined.

Primary closure

Methods of closing wounds

The majority of surgical wounds in children heal by primary intention, which is facilitated by primary closure. The primary aim of wound closure is to restore the physical integrity of the damaged tissue and normal function, with minimum disruption, as quickly as possible (Hollander and Singer, 1999). In addition, it is vital to consider the aesthetic appearance of the wound. Primary closure is achieved by bringing the wound edges together in apposition and adequately securing the edges, so that the natural healing process can occur (Bruns *et al*, 1998). The surface of the wound will usually be totally sealed within 48 hours (Dealey, 1999). The effectiveness of primary closure will depend upon the right choice and correct application of closure materials (Heath, 1998). The ideal wound closure technique should allow for a meticulous closure, be easily and rapidly applied, be painless, of low risk to the healthcare professional using the technique, be inexpensive and result in minimal scarring with a low infection rate (Hollander and Singer, 1999). Sutures, in particular nylon sutures, are the gold standard, due to the favourable cosmetic results, are time honoured and the most commonly used wound closure technique (Hollander and Singer, 1999; Tritle *et al*, 2001). Absorbable sutures should be used primarily for subcuticular tissue closure because of the increased difficulty in achieving a meticulous closure in the epithelial layer, which affects the cosmetic appearance of the wound (Hollander and Singer, 1999). However, rapidly absorbable sutures are widely used for skin closure in children, particularly abdominal wounds, in order to avoid the discomfort associated with suture removal. More recently, tissue adhesives have become an increasingly popular choice for wound closures (Bruns *et al*, 1998). Other alternatives include staples/clips and adhesive tapes/strips. *Table 6.2a* outlines the advantages and disadvantages of the main methods of closing wounds. If a wound is not closed effectively, its tensile strength may not be sufficient to maintain its integrity, with the potential for the wound to dehisce.

Table 6.2a: Methods of closing wounds (Bernard *et al*, 2001; Bruns, 1998; Hollander and Singer, 1999; Osmond *et al*, 1995; Tritle *et al*, 2001)

	Advantages	Disadvantages
Sutures	Gold standard and time honoured. Can achieve meticulous closure with excellent cosmetic results. Greatest tensile strength. Lowest dehiscence rates. Wide choice of materials and application techniques, which can be tailored to each individual wound.	Need to be removed (can be traumatic for children). Greatest tissue reactivity (although newer synthetic materials are less reactive). Highest cost (due to time commitment from healthcare professionals). Slow to apply. High risk of needle stick injuries.
Staples/ clips	Rapid to apply. Cost effective. Low risk of tissue reactivity. Low risk of needle stick injuries. Low cost.	Less able to achieve a meticulous closure which affects cosmetic appearance. May interfere with investigations such as CT MRI scanning. Need to be removed (can be traumatic for children).
Adhesive tapes/ strips	Quick and easy to apply. Cost effective. Provide additional barrier to protect the wound. Minimal tissue reaction. Low infection rates. No risk of needle stick injuries. Low cost. Comfortable and easy to remove.	Requires meticulous application, particularly epithelial edges must be precisely approximated without tension to ensure good cosmetic results. Dehiscence may be a problem, particularly in wounds under higher tension. Frequently become dislodged. Not appropriate for use where hair is present. Not suitable for flexible area, such as joints and hands. May not bath or shower until after removal of the strips.
Tissue adhesive	Useful in minor lacerations as there is no need for local anaesthesia. Potentially eliminates the need for follow visits. Reduces the need for additional procedure to remove suture/clips. Potential good cosmetic outcome in low tension wounds. Excellent for children with needle phobias. Fast to apply. There appears to be minimal tissue reaction with adhesives. Low infection rates. No risk of needle stick injuries. Low cost.	Requires meticulous application; glue on the surface of the wound may hinder epithelialisation. Cosmetic outcome may be inferior to traditional wound dressings. Dehiscence may be a problem, particularly in wounds under higher tension. Limited application, not yet adequately studied in surgical incisional wounds or wounds under high tension. Cost of adhesive more expensive than other methods (however overall cost effective, primarily due to reduced contact time with healthcare professionals).

Management of primary closed wounds

The management of primary closed wounds is straightforward. However, there will be slight differences depending upon type of closure, wound depth, position of the wound and the individual child and family's needs. The initial dressing is applied in theatre; therefore, the type of dressing is usually determined by the surgeon's preference. In practice, this usually consists of an island dressing, such as a self-adhesive low-adherent dressing or a film dressing, with few significant differences between these dressings (*Table 6.1b*) (Dealey, 1999). However, a film dressing allows for early inspection of the wound, whereas a low-adherent dressing will absorb any minor post-operative oozing. From a psychological point of view, some children may prefer to view the wound site, where others may not. Unless there is any indication to do so, such as excessive oozing, or exudate, which may indicate either haemorrhage or infection respectively, there is no need to change dressing daily. Routine swabbing with normal saline is an outdated practice, and potentially exposes the wound to environmental contaminants, traumatising fragile granulating tissue (Dealey, 1999; Gould, 2001). Unnecessary practices cause additional distress to the child and family. Once the wound surface has sealed (usually by 48 hours), the dressing can be removed and need not be replaced.

Removal of the dressing is the ideal opportunity to assess the wound for any abnormalities and ensure that the healing process is continuing appropriately. Observations of the wound include:

- The colour of the wound and tissue in the surrounding area
- Blood loss and evidence of continued oozing
- Temperature of surrounding tissue
- The presence, colour and amount of any exudate on the wound surface and on the dressing
- Swelling.

Removal of the dressing should consider the psychological needs of the child, the assessment of pain, the provision of analgesia, and appropriate preparation and support that will be required by the child and family prior to, during and after the procedure.

In general, normal hygiene routines can be maintained once the dressing has been removed. However, bathing should be avoided if adhesive strips have been used, as prolonged contact with water will loosen their adhesiveness (Hollander and Singer, 1999). Care should be taken with tissue adhesives; again avoid excessive soaking in water or abrasive rubbing, which may dislodge the adhesive (Hollander and Singer, 1999). If sutures or staples are present, they should be checked to make sure that they are intact and the entry sites should be examined for any signs of inflammation. The application of a dressing should be considered, if sutures or staples have been inserted, because of the potential to catch on clothing or be pulled by the inquisitive young child. Drying of the wound can be prevented by the application of white petrolatum (Hollander and Singer, 1999).

The timing of the removal of sutures is a balance between providing the wound edges with support and achieving a good cosmetic result (Castille, 1998). In general, sutures and staples should be removed at about seven days post-operatively, when epithelialisation has occurred. Early removal of facial wounds is recommended at about five days (Castille, 1998), because they heal rapidly due to having a good blood supply. Early removal of sutures minimises the formation of scar tracts at the entry and exit sites of the sutures, improving the cosmetic appearance of the wound (Hollander and Singer, 1999). Sutures in wounds where there is high tension, for example over joints or in hands, should be left longer, i.e. 10–14 days (Castille, 1998; Hollander and Singer, 1999). Staff removing sutures or clips should be familiar with the procedures to remove these in their area of work. Nicol *et al* (2001) provide a detailed description of the principles of the procedures necessary for the removal of sutures, both interrupted and continuous sutures, clips and the application of adhesive strips.

Post-operative haemorrhage

The main complications related to post-operative wounds are haemorrhage, infection, dehiscence, sinus and fistula formation (Dealey, 1999). The two acute complications of haemorrhage and dehiscence are outlined within this section. To prevent repetition infection will be discussed with complex surgical wounds, along with open wounds, sinus and fistula formation.

Some blood loss during surgery is inevitable. Failure to adequately cauterise blood vessels during surgery will result in continued blood loss in the immediate post-operative phase (Dealey, 1999). It is essential that post-operative wound dressings are frequently observed in recovery and on the ward in the immediate post-operative period. Large amounts of blood loss will be rapidly apparent, whereas slow insidious leakage of blood or internal loss may not; therefore, routine checking of wounds should be continued with post-operative observations. Cardiovascular monitoring should be carried out regularly to assist in the early detect of internal bleeding and haemorrhagic shock and is discussed in relation to the post-operative care of the child in *Chapter 4*. Excessive post-operative bleeding may require the application of pressure and a firm dressing and/or exploration of the wound in theatre for ligation of blood vessels. Bleeding will delay wound healing and weaken the wound, and could result in the formation of a haematoma, which will cause pain and is a potential site for infection (Dealey, 1999).

Wound dehiscence

There does not appear to be any available literature in terms of incidence or management of potential post-operative wound complications, such as dehiscence, sinus or fistula formation in children. Wound dehiscence is literally opening or splitting of the wound and can occur in any of the layers of the wound, together or independently. If the deeper muscle layers of the wound dehisce an incisional hernia results, which may not become obvious until months after surgery. Factors which contribute to wound dehiscence include: poor selection of suture material (Hollander and Singer, 1999); inadequate primary closure; type of surgery (for example, dehiscence is more common in abdominal surgery and emergency procedures); early removal of sutures; and the presence of infection (Dealey, 1999). Care will depend upon the extent of the wound breakdown. In general, treatment is conservative, and wound healing is promoted through the appropriate dressing selection and allowing the wound to heal by granulation (Dealey, 1999). Infections must be treated appropriately. Re-suturing may be necessary.

Ongoing care and discharge advice

It is vital that the child and family receive appropriate discharge advice in relation to the ongoing care of the wound. With the increasingly shortening hospital stay, education relating to early wound management and the recognition of signs of inflammation are vital. Although standardised wound care instructions may assist in improving compliance to care and aid in understanding (Casey, 1999; Hollander and Singer, 1999), information must be tailored to each child's needs, and include:

- Pain management

- When to remove dressings (if this is not done prior to discharge or by community nurse)

- Descriptions of signs and symptoms of inflammation

- Bathing/showering instructions (or restrictions): showering is preferable, patting the wound dry, avoiding excessive rubbing, not using talcum powder

- Any limitations to mobility/activities

- Application of moisturisers/white petrolatum

- When to remove adhesive strips, if applicable

- Details of where and when sutures/clips are removed

- Who to contact (this should include contacts for day/night and weekends)

- Details of any referrals that are made to community staff, their role and the expected day and time (if possible) of the visit

- Returning to school.

Primary closure with insertion of a wound drain

Drains allow for any fluid or potential fluid to drain from the base of the wound. They are inserted into wounds, if there is likely to be excessive exudate, blood loss, pus or the presence of body fluids, for example, bile. Although there are many variations in the types of drainage systems, they can generally be divided into two main types (Dealey, 1999):

1. *Open drains:* comprise of a variety of materials, such as tubes, corrugated rubber and ribbon gauze. The type of material will depend on the depth of the wound and type of fluid anticipated. The fluid drains directly onto the dressing, which can be uncomfortable and may require frequent dressing changes (Dealey, 1999). Due to an open channel for bacteria, which can potentially infect the wound bed, infection is a major concern (Dealey, 1999). Therefore, these types of drains are only really suitable for short-term use in wounds where minimal drainage is predicted.

2. *Closed drains:* consist of a tube with islets along the shaft; this end is inserted into the wound with the opposite end connected to a receptacle, which creates a vacuum. The vacuum provides a slight suctioning effect, thereby promoting drainage of the wound bed. There are many types of drainage systems, with some designed to be connected to specifically-designed suction machines providing additional suction.

The decision to insert a drain should not be taken lightly. The balance between the overall benefit and the risks needs to be considered. The greatest risk is increased potential for development of a wound infection (Briggs, 1997). Ideally, drains should be removed after 24–48 hours (Dealey, 1999). The presence of a drain necessitates additional procedures for the child, and removal is an added stress. In addition, drains are usually inserted through a stab wound, and although the site is usually near the main wound, results in an additional wound and scar.

Unfortunately there are few studies relating to the care, management and removal of wound drains (Briggs, 1997). Decisions must involve the multidisciplinary team; in particular, there must be close liaison with the surgeon who inserted the drain. Debate surrounds the methods of removing a drain, in particular vacuum drains (Briggs, 1997). Consensus appears to be to release the vacuum, then apply gentle but continuous traction to remove the drain. There has been a tradition of removing the drain in stages based on the belief that this will promote wound healing from the base of the wound bed, preventing sinus and fistula formation. There does not appear to be any evidence to refute or support this practice.

Complex wounds

Wounds can be classified as chronic because of the underlying aetiology or delayed healing. Chronic wounds are more likely to occur in the elderly and patients with multi-system problems and, although these are often due to pressure (decubitus ulcers), vascular disease (venous ulcers) or cancer cells (fungating lesions), often the reasons and the patho-physiology are unclear (Dealey, 1999). Although not common, chronic wounds do exist in children, but will not be discussed. The management of more complex wounds and potential wound complications will be outlined.

Delayed primary suture and healing by second intention

In wounds where there has been considerable bacterial contamination, for example a large abscess, traumatic injury with an open wound, leakage of body fluid or such intestinal contents that contain bacteria or extensive tissue loss, it may not be possible to close the wound (Dealey, 1999). Two options are delayed primary closure or leaving the wound to heal by second intention.

In delayed primary closure, the wound is closed after about five days, with management aimed at allowing time to treat the complication, such as free drainage of pus and antibiotic therapy to treat infections. The dressing choice should encourage drainage of fluid, keep the open area moist and warm, and ensure minimal discomfort on removal of the dressing *(Table 6.1b)*. Promoting primary granulation is not a major aim, as the wound will subsequently be closed (Dealey, 1999). Delayed primary closure is not possible if there is extensive tissue loss; therefore, leaving the wound to heal by granulation, contraction and epithelialisation (second intention) may be more appropriate (Dealey, 1999). The aim of care will be directed towards promoting granulation and healing without complications, such as infection. The choice of dressing, assessment of the wound at each dressing change and ensuring atraumatic dressing changes are vital.

Selection of dressing in open wounds will depend upon the stage of healing, the position of the wound and the amount of exudate *(Table 6.1b)*. Traditional gauze soaked with antiseptic and packed into the wound is no longer appropriate, as these types of dressings do not promote healing, dry the wound, damage granulation tissue on removal, are painful to remove and require frequent changes (Dealey, 1999). The comfort of the child is paramount. The child and family should be involved in the decision-making process and discussions about the choice of dressings. This requires honest and open dialogue about the relative benefits and disadvantages of the available dressings, including frequency of dressing changes.

An objective assessment and subsequent evaluation are essential if accurate judgements are to be made on the progress of the wound, and to ensure the choice of dressing is appropriate and its effectiveness monitored (Dealey, 1999). The use of an assessment chart should be an integral part of wound care for all complex wounds, and should include information relating to the type of wound, stage of healing, colour, odour and dimensions of the wound; if appropriate, a diagram of the wound and the condition of the surrounding skin. In addition, there should be a record of the dressings that have been used, including dates and summaries of their effectiveness. The ease of removal and comfort of the child should be recorded at each dressing change. Documentation must be of sufficient detail to enable all members of staff to be familiar with the wound and treatment regimes. Poor documentation and a lack of understanding of the stages of wound healing have been identified as a contributing factor to the lack of continuity in the management of wounds (Dealey, 1999).

Wound infection

Despite increased understanding about the spread of infection and standards in maintaining asepsis, post-operative wound infection remains a significant post-operative complication (Emmerson *et al*, 1996; Plowman *et al*, 1999; Reilly *et al*, 2001). Therefore, the prevention of infection needs to be a priority for all healthcare professionals and in all healthcare settings. This includes understanding and adhering to policies in relation to universal infection control precautions (Bolyard *et al*, 1998; Gould, 1997; Xavier 1999). These include:

- Appropriate hand washing
- Correct disposal of waste (including sharps) and linen
- Wearing gloves and a plastic apron whenever contact with blood or body fluids is anticipated.

The spread of bacteria via hands is well established and hand washing had been implicated as the single most important procedure in preventing the spread of infection (Bolyard *et al*, 1998; Bree-Williams and Waterman, 1996; Gould, 1997; Gould and Chamberlain, 1997; Xavier, 1999). Effective hand washing, and its role in reducing the spread of infection, is the cornerstone of efforts to reduce cross-infection (Gould, 1997).

In addition to universal infection control precautions, more specific clinical techniques should be used when an invasive procedure is performed. Asepsis is the prevention of microbial contamination of living tissue by excluding, removing or killing micro-organisms (Xavier, 1999). The aim of performing an aseptic technique is to prevent the spread of infection to a susceptible patient, by direct or indirect means (Xavier, 1999). This would include preventing the transmission of micro-organisms into a healthy wound (Bree-Williams and Waterman, 1996). Maintaining a meticulous aseptic technique when undertaking wound care will minimise the risk of cross-infection between patients.

There appears to be much confusion among nursing staff in relation to undertaking an aseptic technique (Bree-Williams and Waterman, 1996; Hallett, 2000). This has been fuelled by adherence to ritualistic practices (Bree-Williams and Waterman, 1996; Hollingworth, 1998), which have not reflected sound principles and are often based on local historical practices, the change in designs of dressing packs (Bree-Williams and Waterman, 1996), and lack of training packages to support the education of nurses (Bree-Williams and Waterman, 1996; Gould and Chamberlain, 1997). Furthermore, aseptic technique procedures vary from one hospital to another. The principles that underpin standardised procedures should be justifiable and regularly take full account of recent and relevant research. There is little empirical evidence to categorically prove that aseptic techniques reduce the incidence of wound infection (Bree-Williams and Waterman, 1996; Gould and Chamberlain, 1997). Questions have been raised as to whether this practice is necessary (Bree-Williams and Waterman, 1996; Gould and Chamberlain, 1997; Hallettt, 2000; Meers *et al*, 1997), particularly for chronic wounds (Baxter 2002). However, the general consensus is that a sterile technique should be used to dress open wounds. Xavier (1999) provides a useful review of the principles of undertaking an aseptic technique.

In common with aseptic technique, there is much confusion relating to the cleansing of wounds. Firstly, not all wounds require routine cleaning. However, infected and contaminated wounds will require cleaning to remove any debris that might hinder the healing process (Towler, 2001). Current consensus opinion in relation to cleansing wound includes:

- Avoiding direct swabbing because of the trauma caused to the wound bed

- Irrigation with normal saline is current method of choice.

(Towler, 2001)

The four cardinal signs and symptoms of infection are redness in the tissue surrounding the wound, heat, pain and swelling. A systemic rise in temperature may be the first sign if infection develops in deeper tissues. Other indicators that may indicate the presence of a wound infection include :

- Wound healing is not progressing at the expected rate
- Discharge/increased exudate or changes in the exudate, such as colour, smell and texture
- Discolouration of the wound bed

- Cellulitis
- Granulation tissue which remains friable and continues to bleed
- Unexpected pain, tenderness or throbbing
- Puckering at the base of the wound
- Breakdown of a previously healthy wound.

(Cutting and Harding, 1994; Gould, 2001)

Most wounds are colonised with bacteria (Dealey, 1999). Although a wound swab is necessary to determine the type of bacteria, it does not prove an infection is present. Laboratory findings should be combined with a clinical evaluation of the wound, with treatment only commencing if there are clinical indications that an infection is present (Dealey, 1999; Gould, 2001). The bacteria most commonly associated with post-operative wound infections are *Staphylococci*, *Gram-negative rods* and *Streptococci* (Gould, 2001). *Table 6.2b* provides an overview of these bacteria. Many bacteria that have the potential to cause wound infections (*Table 6.2b*) are part of the normal flora of healthy individuals, including healthcare workers. In addition, *Gram-negative* bacteria thrive in warm damp environments, where there is little organic material (Gould, 2001). It is therefore essential that universal precautions, such as keeping the environment clean and well-ventilated, appropriate storage of equipment, and meticulous hand hygiene, are maintained.

The management of an infected wound will include a combination of systemic antibiotics, the use of topical agents and choosing the most appropriate dressing. The treatment options will depend upon causative organisms and assessment of the wound, in particular type of exudates. The management of resistant strains of organisms such as methicillin-resistant *Staphylococcus aureus* (MRSA) is particularly difficult and it is vital that these infections are managed appropriately. Controlling the spread of MRSA is vital because treatments are expensive and is associated with poor recovery rates (Morrison and Stolarek, 2000). Local guidelines and policies in relation to the management of MRSA should include the principles outlined in the

British Society for Antimicrobial Chemotherapy, the Hospital Infection Society and the Infection Control Nurses Association's (1998) guidelines.

Table 6.2b: Overview of bacteria associated with surgical wounds (Gould, 2001)

Bacteria	Strain	Characteristics
Staphylococcus A group of Gram-positive bacteria and are a major cause of hospital-acquired infections. They are a major concern because of the evolution of resistant strains.	*Staphylococcus aureus*	Forms part of the normal flora of the nose, throat, axillae and perineum of many individuals. Transmission to a vulnerable individual can result in infection. A major source of hospital acquired infections including wound infections.
	methicillin-resistant *Staphylococcuss aureus* (MRSA)	A resistant strain of *Staphylococcus aureus* which evolved as a result of careless prescription of antibiotics and lack of attention to infection control policies and procedures. Carriers develop in the same way as they do for *Staphylococcus aureus*. MRSA is difficult to eradicate.
	Staphylococcus epidermidis	Less virulent than *Staphylococcus aureus*; however, the bacteria adhere to plastic and metal devices, therefore are a potential cause of concern where prosthetic devices are used.
Gram-negative Rods A broad group of bacteria, including the anaerobic bacteria of the gut.	*Escherchia coli Serratia Klebseilla*	Commensal organism living in the human gut. Can cause serious infections and is a potential pathogen in wound infections, where there has been surgery on the intestinal tract.
Streptococcus Chain forming *Gram-positive cocci*; Can cause serious infectious outbreaks due the bacteria being carried asymptomatically in healthy people. In general remain sensitive to penicillin, although there is increasing evidence to suggest penicillin-resistant strains are developing.	*Streptococcus pyrogenes*	Of the *Streptococcus* group this is the most likely to be responsible for wound infections and includes the sub group, *Group A beta haemolytic Streptococci* which can have serious consequences. The bacteria are carried in the nasopharynx and dispersed by droplets.
	Streptococcus pneumoniae	A commensal organism living harmlessly in the respiratory tract. Causes acute infections in susceptible individuals such as otitis media, pneumonia and meningitis, Not usually associated with wound infection.
	Streptococcus faecalis	Commensal organism living in the human gut. Can cause serious infections and is a potential pathogen in wound infections, where there has been surgery on the intestinal tract.

Sinus and fistula formation

A sinus is a tract from an abscess or cavity to the skin surface. Treatment options include: surgical incision and leaving open the sinus, or insertion of a drain that allows drainage of fluid (Dealey, 1999). A fistula is a tract formed between one organ to another or to the skin surface, usually in the abdomen and develops spontaneously following surgery (Dealey, 1999). Although a fistula may close spontaneously, the majority require surgical intervention. Wound care around the fistula site is important, as fluid leakage can cause excoriation of the surrounding tissue, particularly if this is faecal fluid.

Wound hypertrophy and keloid scars

Although the healing process can take up to one year to complete (Moore and Foster, 2002; Russell, 2002) (*Table 6.1a*), most wounds are remoulded and form a smooth flat surface (Dealey, 1999). Wound healing processes that are not well controlled can result in excessive deposition of collagen in the final stages of healing, resulting in hypertrophic and keloid scars. These scars are raised, erythematous, hard and may cause pruritus (Poston, 2000). With hypertrophic scars, the excessive collagen deposition remains within the wound margins; in keloid scars, there is excessive collagen deposition in the areas surrounding the scar (Poston, 2000). Treatments for both are difficult and not always successful and include surgical excision, intralesional steroids, laser therapy, ultrasound and cryotherapy (Poston, 2000). Less invasive management includes cosmetic camouflage, compression therapy and the application of silicon gel sheeting (Poston, 2000).

Scar massage is one of the management strategies used within burns rehabilitation in order to minimise the hypertrophy of scars and reduce pruritus and pain (Field *et al*, 2000, Rochet and Zaouri, 2002). The techniques involve massaging an emollient into the wound using circular movements.

Meeting the holistic needs of the child and family

Any surgical procedure that has resulted in an incisional wound will cause pain, due to the inflammatory response, damaged nerve cells and enhanced pain sensations in the damaged tissue and surrounding area (Fitzgerald and Howard, 2003). It is therefore vital that all children with an acute surgical wound have their pain assessed and managed appropriately (*Chapter 5*). Unfortunately, procedural related pain, which includes wound dressing changes, has not always been a high priority in the care of children (Yaster *et al*, 2003). Analgesic, sedation (or general anaesthesia), distraction techniques (Harper and Kleiber, 1999) are all important considerations. It is important that the first dressings change is not traumatic, particularly if it is anticipated that there will be regular dressing changes over a long period. Preparation should be appropriate for the age and stage of development of the child, and the type of procedure being performed (Casey, 1999). Depending upon the age and stage of development of the child, preparation through the use of play and the involvement of a play therapist are invaluable (Chandler, 1994; Ellerton and Merriam, 1994).

The child and family should be involved in the decision-making process. If repeated dressings are required, it is essential that there is open and honest dialogue about the relative benefits and disadvantages of the available dressings, including frequency of dressing changes. This will assist the child and family to participate in discussions about the choice of dressings. Although procedures, such as suture removal, should not be painful (Nicol *et al*, 2001), they can be anxiety-provoking for the child, who may anticipate pain or discomfort. Nicol *et al* suggest that adequate preparation can reduce anxiety and correct positioning will minimise any discomfort. Certainly a child who is motionless will make any procedure technically easier (Selbst and Zempsky, 2003). However, caution should always be used when restraining a child, and appropriate guidelines, such as those published by the Royal College of Nursing (2003), should be adopted (*Chapter 2*).

References

Baxter H (2001) How a discipline came of age: a history of wound care. *J Wound Care* 11(10): 383–92

Bree-Williams FJ, Waterman H (1996) An examination of nurses' practices while performing aseptic technique. *J Adv Nurs* 23(1): 48–56

Bernard L, Friedlander SF, Eichenfield LF *et al* (2001) A prospective comparison of Octyl Cynoacrylate tissue adhesive (Dermabond) and suture material for the closure of excisional wounds in children and adolescents. *Arch Dermatol* 137(9): 1177–80

Bolyard EA, Tablan OC, Williams WW *et al* (1998) Guidelines for infection control in healthcare personnel. *Infect Contr Hosp Epidemiol* 19: 407–63

Briggs M (1997) Principles of closed surgical wound care. *J Wound Care* 6(6): 288–92

British Society for Antimicrobial Chemotherapy, Hospital Infection Society and the Infection Control Nurses Association Combined Working Party (1998) Revised guidelines for the control of *methicillin-resistant Staphylococcus aureus* infections in hospitals. *J Hosp Infect* 39(4): 253–90

Bruns TB, Robinson BS, Smith RJ *et al* (1998) A new tissue adhesive for laceration repair in children. *J Pediatrics* 132 (6): 1067–70

Casey G (2001) Wound dressings. *Pediatr Nurs* 13(4): 39–42

Casey G (1999) Wound management in children. *Emerg Nurse* 7(6): 33–39

Casey G (1998) Wound healing. *Primary HealthCare* 8(10): 31–36

Castille K (1998) Suturing. *Nurs Stand* 12(41): 41–48

Chandler K (1994) Play preparation for surgery. *Surgical Nurse* 7(4): 14–16

Cutting K, Harding KG (1994) Criteria for identifying wound infection. *J Wound Care* 3(4): 198–201

Dealey C (1999) *The Care of Wounds: A Guide for Nurses,* 2nd edn. Blackwell Science, London

Doig CM, Wilkinson AW (1976) Wound infections in a children's hospital. *Br J Surgery* 63: 647–50

Ellerton ML, Merriam C (1994) Preparing children and families psychologically for day surgery: an evaluation. *J Adv Nurs* 19(6): 1057–62

Emmerson AM, Enstone JE, Griffin M *et al* (1996) The second national prevalence survey of infection in hospitals: overview and results. *J Hosp Infect* 32: 175–90

Field T, Peck M, Hernandez-Reif M *et al* (2000) Postburn itching, pain, and psychological symptoms are reduced with massage therapy. *J Burn Care Rehab* **21**(3): 189–93

Fitzgerald M, Howard F (2003) The neurobiological basis of pediatric pain. In: Schechter NL, Berde CB, Yaster M, eds. *Pain in Infants, Children and Adolescents*. Lippincott, Williams and Wilkins, USA

Gibson F, Bamford O (2001) Focus group interventions to examine the role and development of clinical nurse specialist. *J Nurs Man* **9**: 331–42

Gould D (2001) Clean surgical wounds: prevention of infection. *Nurs Stand* **15**(49): 45–52

Gould D (1997) *Hand Care Monitoring Standards. Hygienic Hand Decontamination*. Macmillan Magazines, London

Gould D, Chamberlain A (1997) The use of a ward-based educational teaching package to enhance nurses' compliance with infection control policies. *J Clin Nurs* **6**(1): 55–67

Gray D, Cooper P (2001) Nutrition and wound healing: what is the link? *J Wound Care* **10**(3): 86–89.

Hallettt C (2000) Infection control in wound care: a study of fatalism in community nursing. *J Clin Nurs* **9**(1): 103–109

Harker J (2001) Role of the nurse consultant in tissue viability. *Nurs Stand* **15**(49): 39–42

Harper D, Kleiber C (1999) Effects of distraction on children's pain and distress during medical procedures: a meta-analysis. *Nurs Res* **48**(1): 44–49

Heath S (1998) *Perioperative Care of the Child*. Mark Allen Publishing Ltd, Salisbury

Hollander JE, Singer AJ (1999) Laceration management. *Ann Emerg Med* **34**(3): 356–67

Hollingworth H (1998) Using a non-sterile technique in wound care. *Profess Nurse* **13**(4): 226–29

Horwitz J, Chawals W, Doski J *et al* (1998) Pediatric wound infections: a prospective multicentre study. *Ann Surgery* **227**(4): 553–58

House of Commons Health Select Committee (1997) *Hospital Services for Children and Young People: Fifth Report*. Stationery Office, London

Lait ME, Smith LN (1998) Wound management: a literature review. *J Clin Nurs* **7**(1): 11–17

Meers P, McPherson M, Sedgwick J (1997) *Infection Control in Healthcare*, 2nd edn. Stanley Thornes, Cheltenham

Moore P, Foster L (2002) Acute surgical wound care 1: an overview of treatment. In: White R, Harding K, eds. *Trends in Wound Care*. Quay Books, Bath

Morison M, Moffat C, Bridel-Nixon J *et al* (1997) *Nursing Management of Chronic Wounds*, 2nd edn. Mosby, London

Morrison L, Stolarek I (2000) Does MRSA affect patient outcomes in the elderly? A retrospective pilot study. *J Hosp Infect* 45(2): 169–71

Nichols RL (1998) Post-operative wound infections in the age of drug-resistant Gram positive bacteria. *Am J Med* 104 (5A): 11S–16S

Nicol M, Bavin C, Bedford-Turner S *et al* (2001) Wound assessment: removal of skin sutures. *Nurs Stand* 16(8): 39–42

Osmond MH, Klassen TP, Quinn JV (1995) Economic comparison of a tissue adhesive and suturing in the repair of pediatric facial lacerations. *J Pediatrics* 126 (6): 892–95

Parker L (2000) Applying the principles of infection control to wound care. *Br J Nurs* 9(7): 398–404

Plowman R, Roberts JA, Groves N *et al* (1999) *The Socioeconomic Burden of Hospital-Acquired Infection*. Public Health Laboratory Service, London

Poston J (2000) The use of silicone gel sheeting in the management of hypertrophic and keloid scars. *J Wound Care* 9(9): 10–16

Reilly J, Baird D, Hill R (2001) The importance of definitions and methods in surgical wound infection audit. *J Hosp Infect* 47(1): 64–66

Rochet Jm, Zaouri A (2002) Burn scars: rehabilitation and skin care. *Revue du Practicien*. 52(20): 2258–63

Royal College of Nursing (2003) *Restraining, Holding Still and Containing Children and Young People*. RCN, London

Russell L (2002) Understanding of wound healing and how dressings help. In: White R, Harding K eds. *Trends in Wound Care*. Quay Books, Bath

Selbst SM, Zempsky WT (2003) Sedation and analgesia in the emergency department. In: Schechter NL, Berde CB, Yaster M, eds. *Pain in Infants, Children and Adolescents*. Lippincott, Williams and Wilkins, USA

Shipperley T, Martin C (2002) The physiology of wound healing: an emergency response. *Nurs Times* 98(8): 54–55

Towler J (2001) Cleansing traumatic wounds with swabs, water or saline. *J Wound Care* 10(6): 231–34

Tritle N, Haller J, Gray S (2001) Aesthetic comparison of wound closure techniques in a porcine model. *Laryngoscope* 111(11): 1949–51

Watret L, White R (2001) Surgical wound management: the role of dressings. *Nurs Stand* 15(44): 59–69

White R, Cooper R, Kingsley A (2002) A topical issue: the use of antibacterials in wound pathogen control. In: White R, Harding K, eds. *Trends in Wound Care*. Quay Books, Bath

Xavier G (1999) Asepsis. *Nurs Stand* 13(36): 49–53

Yaster M, Tobin JR,Kost-Byerly S (2003) Local anesthetics. In: Schechter NL, Berde CB, Yaster M, eds. *Pain in Infants, Children and Adolescents*. Lippincott, Williams and Wilkins, USA

SEVEN

MINIMISING THE EFFECTS OF HOSPITALISATION IN CHILDREN

Reducing the negative impact of hospitalisation upon the child was clearly stated within *The Welfare of Children and Young People in Hospital* document:

> '*children are admitted to hospital only if the care they require cannot be as well provided at home, in a day clinic or on a day basis in hospital*'
>
> (Department of Health, 1991: 2).

The initial drive towards reducing hospital admissions was to minimise the effects of hospitalisation in children. However, containing healthcare costs by reducing inpatient admissions has proved to be attractive to governments facing escalating healthcare costs (Glasper and Lowson, 1998; Turner, 1998). The cost burden is often moved to the primary care setting (Bridger and Rees, 1995) and, unfortunately, resources have not necessarily reflected changes in service provision.

New technologies, a growing evidence-base upon which to underpin treatments, societal changes, including increased consumerism, escalating costs, changing professional boundaries, demographic changes, and changing patterns of diseases contribute to the need to develop new ways of working. Within the last decade, ambulatory care has become the fastest growing branch of healthcare in Western societies (Glasper and Lowson, 1998) and, in its broadest concept, describes the provision of healthcare that does not require an overnight stay in hospital (Turner, 1998). Ambulatory care is an umbrella term and includes services such as: day care, telecare (the provision of information by telephone), expanding practice within accident and emergency departments, expanding practice and services within health centres, expanding practice within outpatients departments, specialist outreach services, and community services.

This chapter will consider the effects hospitalisation may have on children, both in terms of the child's initial reaction to hospitalisation and the potential long-term effects upon development. The specific role of day care and continuing care in the community as ways of reducing inpatient stays for children, who have had a surgical procedure, will be outlined.

7.1 Effects of hospitalisation

Childhood experiences have a profound effect upon the developing child (Taylor *et al*, 1999). Healthcare professionals need to have an understanding of the potential effects that healthcare interventions and hospitalisation have upon the child and family, in order to minimise these effects and enhance the potential positive effects of these experiences. Unfortunately, the psychological needs of children have not always been a priority within the healthcare setting (Taylor *et al*, 1999). The *Curtis Report* (Ministry of Health, 1946) claimed that the most damaging elements characterising the lives of young children were separation from the family and an unfamiliar environment. Within the UK, John Bowlby and James Robertson, colleagues in child psychiatry, led the research conducted in the 1950s, which related to the experiences of young children and the effects of hospitalisation upon children, particularly focusing upon the separation of the child from his/her parents. The influence of their work cannot be underestimated and was certainly reflected in government reports relating to the welfare of children in hospital at the time, most noticeably the *Platt Report* (Ministry of Health, 1959). Alsop-Shields and Mohay (2001) provide an insightful review of their work, theories and continuing influence upon childcare practices.

Bowlby, commissioned by the World Health Organization, reported on the effects of separation of children from their carers following reviews of individual cases, children in orphanages and animal studies. This work culminated in the publication of *Maternal Care and Mental Health* (Bowlby, 1951) and suggested that if a child was not permitted to form an affectionate bond with its mother, it would develop an 'affectionless psychopathy'. The child would not develop the ability to feel emotion for anybody else and would have a lack of interest in anybody else's welfare, and that lack of a mother or mother substitute could result in delinquent behaviour in later life. This was reiterated in his later work, in which he suggested that there was a strong causal relationship between the ability to make affectionate bonds, and the later development of neurotic symptoms and personality disorders (Bowlby, 1979). Interpreters of Bowlby's work have assumed this to mean full-time mothering. Criticisms of his early research have included: its lack of methodological rigour (choice of children and the biases within control groups), sweeping statements not substantiated within the data, conclusions that cannot be attributed to the lack of a maternal presence alone (primarily, the environments that many of these children experienced were far from ideal, lacking in resources, stimulation, and the provision of basic physical care) and failure to test his hypothesis (Alsop-Shields and Mohay, 2001; Clarke and Clarke, 1976; Rutter, 1972; Taylor *et al*, 1999). Attachment theories are a way of conceptualising the ability of human beings to make strong bonds with others, and understand the emotional distress and personality disturbances, including: anxiety, anger, depression and emotional detachment, which may be a result of separation or loss (Bowlby, 1979).

An understanding of the stages through which a child develops attachments is important to professionals working with children, so that they can minimise disruption to normal development and identify opportunities to maintain or encourage child-parent attachments. Infants pass through several stages as they begin to develop social ties; asocial phase (0–6 weeks), indiscriminate attachments (six weeks to seven months), specific attachments (from about seven months) and multiple attachments (from about 18 months) (Schaffer and Emerson, 1964). These stages have been expanded and redefined:

- *Pre-attachment phase* (six weeks to three months): from about six weeks, babies begin to develop an attraction to other human beings in preference to inanimate objects and engage in social behaviours, such as nestling, gurgling and smiling, which will be displayed to just about anyone, hence the term the social smile

- *Indiscriminate attachment phase* (3–7 months): the social smile disappears and, at about three months, the infant can distinguish between familiar and unfamiliar individuals. Infants will allow strangers to care for them, if this is done to a satisfactory standard

- *Discriminate attachment phase* (7–9 months): typically, the infant develops specific attachments and becomes distressed if separated from the main caregiver; the infant actively seeks the proximity of certain people. Separation protest may also be seen and there may be fear of strangers (lasting through the 8–12 months stage)

- *Multiple attachment phase* (9 months onwards): the infant may become increasingly independent from caregivers and forms attachments with others; however, the strongest attachment will remain with the main caregiver. The 12-month-old prefers to remain within sight of the carer using him/her as a safe base and turning to him/her for comfort, with the 2–3 year old widening his/her exploration field.

(Ainsworth *et al*, 1978)

Ainsworth *et al* developed and tested attachment theories using the strange situation scenario, a systematic approach used to observing a child's behaviours in response to the presence of a parent, stranger or both. This work resulted in the classification of the child's responses into three groups:

- Anxious avoidance/detached

- Anxious resistant/ambivalent

- Securely attached.

Mothers of securely attached infants were identified as being more supportive of their infant's independent play, more sensitive to their needs and more emotionally expressive towards their infants. However, the classifications may merely be observations of temperament and may not demonstrate relationship of child-parent attachment. Thomas and Chess (1977) suggest that, by observing children (using dimensions of temperament), the disposition of the child can be identified and this will affect the attachment process:

- *The easy child:* approaches new events positively, eats well, sleeps well, has regular elimination, is usually happy, adapts to change easily, and is responsive to stimulation

- *The difficult child:* is slow to develop a regular pattern in relation to eating and sleeping, shows negative reactions to new things and changes, often cries and is irritable and is highly responsive to stimuli, for example, reacts vigorously and often negatively to a new food and may spit it out and scream

- *The slow to warm up child:* although not as negative as the difficult child, may show a passive resistance, for instance, when a new food is introduced he may not chew it, but suck it and drool without swallowing, then mildly resist further mouthfuls. Does not show intense reactions, either positive or negative, yet his adaptation although slow, is eventually positive.

Although there are many factors that contribute to the development of secure attachments in infancy and early childhood, it has been estimated that approximately a third of all children are insecure (Bar-Haim *et al*, 2000). This has the potential to place many children at a disadvantage because the child who is secure develops in almost every way faster than the child who is insecure (Shaffer, 2002). Secure toddlers have a longer attention span and are more confident, having more mature and complex play patterns.

These early studies supported the development of hospital practices, such as recognising that the care delivered must be appropriate to each child's developmental stage, and supported the presence of the main carer to be with his/her child. However, the sometimes-overzealous interpretations of these early studies is a potential cause of distress for those parents struggling to form attachments with their child, unable to stay with their child during hospitalisation, and because of the growing use of day nurseries for working mothers. The effects of separation upon subsequent development were reassessed by Rutter (1981; 1972). The important factors for developing secure attachments are:

- A loving relationship
- An unbroken relationship, which is not the same as transient separations
- Stimulating interactions
- Intransient separations, the consistency and quality of care that is important.

(Rutter, 1981; 1972)

Short-term responses to separation, manifested by acute distress, need to be differentiated from the potential effects of long-term separation. The potential long-term effects of not developing a secure attachment in infancy could include:

- Delinquency
- Affectionless psychopathy
- Developmental problems in areas, such as language and cognitive development
- Poor physical growth
- Depression in later life
- Social disinhibition
- Indiscriminate friendships and the inability to form lasting relationships.

(Rutter, 1981; 1972)

These problems have been supported in more recent studies (Teichman *et al*, 1986; Waters *et al*, 2000). There appears to be a significant relationship between the child experiencing parental loss, abuse or serious illness and a change in the attachment classification (Waters *et al*, 2000). This may not be true in every child as there are many interlinking factors that influence development (Taylor *et al*, 1999). The child's emotional reactions to hospitalisation are determined by the interrelationship of personal (natural anxiety traits), interpersonal (maternal anxiety) and environmental factors (day care or inpatient) (Teichman *et al*, 1986). Douglas (1975) conducted a long-term study collecting information on hospital admissions, educational progress, behaviour, parental attitudes and home circumstances, over a 26-year period. The results suggested:

- A single admission to hospital of more than one week duration or repeated admissions (particularly between the ages of six months and five years) are associated with an increase in behavioural disturbances, such as a child who is nervous, difficult to handle, suffers sleep disturbances, loss of bladder control, eating difficulties and stammer

- Some of these behaviours persist into adolescence, particularly nervous tendencies and troublesome behaviour, identified by disruption in the classroom, more delinquent behaviour, unstable job patterns, poor readers and poor concentration

- The vast majority of children show no changes following short duration admissions of less then one week; about one fifth of children may have temporary behavioural changes, with about one tenth showing improved behaviours, such as general improvements, eating better, more talkative, improved speech and lively.

Dissociative disorders in adults correlate highly with childhood trauma (such as subjected to, or witnessing abuse), early separation from a parent and parental dysfunction (Draijer and Langland, 1999).

Caution is needed when interpreting early studies, in that the context in which the data was collected reflected hospital environments and practices in operation at the time. The collective evidence would suggest that the long-term effects of not forming attachments and the impact of separation upon attachments already formed, including prolonged hospitalisation, have the potential to influence a child's long-term development negatively, particular his/her mental well-being. The risks of disturbed behaviour following admission to hospital at an early age could be reduced if children who are highly dependent on their mothers, known to be under stress at home, or experience excessive sibling rivalry, were treated at home or, if hospitalisation was necessary, had their treatment postponed (Douglas, 1975). In addition to the long-term effects of hospitalisation, there are the short-term effects a child may experience during hospital stay or in the immediate period post discharge.

The most visible effects a child displays when separated from his/her carers occur during the discriminate attachment phase (7–9 months). The separation anxiety process was particularly well documented by Robertson (1970; 1958; 1955), who described three typical stages through which an infant progresses when he/she is distressed:

- *Protest:* the infant cries, is inwardly angry and fearful, seeks an attachment figure and can usually be comforted

- *Despair:* the infant appears outwardly calmer, apathetic, does not seek an attachment figure. Self-satisfying behaviours may develop, such as thumb sucking and rocking

- *Detachment:* if the situation continues, the infant may appear to be coping, but generally has given up hope and stops trying to form relationships. The infant may reject the main caregiver when he/she returns.

There is a lack of primary research studies relating solely to the effects of hospitalisation in children, because of inherent difficulties in studying the effects of hospitalisation and its impact upon development in isolation, ethical difficulties in obtaining comparison groups, and changing hospital policies, such as shorter stay and parental participation in care. In fact, the primary sources identified in Sheldon's (1997) recent review of the literature relating to the effects of hospitalisation on children, were primarily drawn from the 1960s and 1970s. Early studies can be of value; firstly, by acting as a reminder as to the reason for changes, and secondly, as a driver for continuing to work towards improving the quality of care and environment for children in hospital, particularly where practice has stagnated.

The vast improvement in hospital environments and working practices, including play and educational facilities, over the latter half of the twentieth century have contributed to a reduction in psychological trauma for older children. In all probability, these changes probably do not compensate for the absence of familiar carer and the subsequent distress experienced by the young child (Sheldon, 1997). Children under three years of age and the majority of children under five years of age exhibit varying degrees of stress during hospitalisation, with many exhibiting behavioural changes in the immediate discharge period (Douglas, 1975; Vernon *et al*, 1965).

Visintainer and Wolfer (1975) measured children's emotional stress and co-operation during five common situations experienced by the child prior to surgery; admission examination, blood testing, pre-operative medication, transport to theatre, and the waiting period in theatre prior to the administration of anaesthesia. All the children studied showed varying degrees of upset. However, children under six years of age were more upset and showed less co-operation. They suggested the most worrying elements of hospital for children were: fear of physical harm or body injury (with its associated counterparts, such as pain, mutilation or death), separation from parents, strange or unknown situations, uncertainties about expected behaviours, and loss of control. Hawthorn's (1974) research, although not purely focusing upon the effects of hospitalisation, highlighted a fundamental lack of knowledge concerning a child's emotional needs while in hospital, with many children spending a high percentage of time on their own, feeling fearful and miserable. Vernon *et al* (1965) found that following discharge children who had an inpatient stay of one week or more were anxious, particularly if parents tried to leave them, had disturbed sleep and demonstrated aggressive behaviours.

Factors which contribute to the experience of an individual child during hospitalisation, include:

- Natural anxiety traits, maternal anxiety and the hospital setting (Teichman *et al*, 1986)

- Parents' presence and length of stay (Robertson, 1970)

- Recent changes in life events unrelated to the hospital admission, such as birth of a sibling, death of a pet, house move, new school or family disruption (Crocker, 1980; Douglas, 1975)

- Negative previous experiences (Vernon *et al*, 1965)
- The severity of the illness.

Practical suggestions for reducing stress experienced by children in hospital include :

- Unrestricted visiting for parents
- Reducing inpatient stay wherever possible
- Establishing whether other distressing events are having a profound effect upon the child and considering ways to help support the child, including the possibility of delaying admission
- Preparing the child and family for the hospital stay
- Exploring previous negative experiences relating to hospitalisation and offering sensitive and appropriate advice to reassure the child and family about the forthcoming admission
- Ensuring first impressions are positive by welcoming the child and family and that admission procedures are informative (for both the family and staff) and reassuring
- Ensuring support is provided, and information giving and reassurance are continued at each step in the hospital stay
- Spending time with the child and family and encouraging them to discuss their anxieties
- Paying attention to detail (often small things make a big difference); making the stay personal by encouraging familiar items from home and remembering the child's interests and dislikes, and incorporating these into care
- Improving hospital environments, which can be frightening, by reducing the clinical appearance of the environment and, if equipment must be visible, ensuring the child and family are aware of its use
- Ensuring there are suitable play and educational facilities, and that the child and family are offered advice on the role

of play and education in the hospital environment as well as the reason for any restrictions

- Ensuring systems of delivering care are reviewed regularly and that the child and family are central by maximising consistency of care, which may include how staff are allocated the children they care for, named/key worker systems, shared beliefs and philosophies of all members of the healthcare team

- Ensuring hospital procedures, policies and guidelines reflect the unique need of the child and family, and that staff implement them consistently.

(Taylor *et al*, 1999)

Despite improvements in facilities for children and their families, the most recent national audit of child health provisions in hospital within the UK (Audit Commission, 1993), although now nearly ten years old, suggests facilities remain patchy. Facilities for parents to stay overnight are limited; there are inadequate numbers of children's nurses, both providing direct clinical care and in management positions, and there is a lack of overall specific guidelines that address children's needs, potentially compromising the quality of the care delivered to children.

7.2 Psychological preparation of children prior to surgery

The child and family may have many misconceptions in relation to hospital routines and medical procedures (Taylor *et al*, 1999). Shorter hospital stays, increased throughput of children and the increased use of day care is reducing the time available to prepare the child and family, both physically and psychologically, for their hospital experience on admission (Carpenter, 1998; Ellerton and Merriam, 1994). This places an increased responsibility upon parents in preparing their child for surgery (Carpenter, 1998). It is essential that every opportunity is utilised to ensure the child and family are sufficiently prepared for the hospital experience. Effective preparation has the potential to reduce the stress and fear of the imminent hospital admission and proposed surgery (Ellerton and Merriam, 1994; LaMontagne *et al*, 1996). The need to adequately prepare children for surgery has been a key feature in policy documents and practice guidelines, such as *Just for the Day* (Thornes, 1991) and *Setting Standards for Children Undergoing Surgery* (Hogg, 1994), and includes preparation prior to admission and throughout the hospital stay, and continuing support following discharge. The nature of the admission may determine the type of preparation. In the case of children admitted for elective surgery from a waiting list, there should be opportunity to prepare children in a more structured setting. Taylor *et al* (1999) suggest three factors that need to be considered in relation to preparing children for hospital, namely: why, how and who?

Early studies exploring children's experiences and perceptions of hospitalisation suggest children have many fears, apprehension, anxieties and misconceptions relating to hospitals, medical procedures, and the role of healthcare professionals (Eiser and Patterson, 1984; Goodman and Adams, 1989; Miron, 1990; Price, 1988; Rodin, 1983). These include:

● Fear of medicines and, in particular, the association with needles and injections

● Fear of medical procedures, such as blood taking, insertion of stitches and operations

● Apprehensi onabout sights and smells, such as disinfectants, blood

● Fear of pain

● Concern about the environment and facilities, such as sleeping and washing facilities and a lack of privacy, unfamiliar food, loss of contact with friends and family, loss of independence.

Recent studies have focused upon factors that contribute to the child's (and the family's) pre-operative anxiety and coping mechanisms, and subsequent behavioural changes (Kain *et al*, 1996; LaMontagne *et al*, 1996; Shirley *et al*, 1998). Factors that contribute to the pre-operative anxiety of children include:

- Anxiety of the mother
- Temperament of the child
- Age of the child
- Quality of previous medical encounters, including previous surgery
- Lack of involvement in pre-operative preparation programmes, particularly if the child is unaware of the reason for being in hospital.

(Kain *et al*, 1996)

Although anxiety is a normal phenomenon in response to a stressful situation, anxiety may be compounded in children because of the child's limited cognitive ability, resulting in misinterpretation and distorting of information. Information must be presented to a child in a format and at a level appropriate to his/her developmental stage level. Lack of prior experiences makes it difficult for the child to assimilate information and integrate new experiences with previous knowledge and therefore predict the outcome of medical interventions. The prevalence of extreme levels of pre-operative anxiety in children has been estimated to be between 40 and 60 percent (Kain *et al*, 1996). In addition, 42 percent of parents demonstrate extreme anxiety, approaching a pathological disorder, prior to their child's surgery (Shirley *et al*, 1998). Factors relating to parental anxiety included the actual surgical and anaesthetic techniques, pre-operative procedures, such as fasting, the potential for the child to experience post-operative pain, and the actual hospital stay (Shirley *et al*, 1998). Anxiety appears to be at the highest level in the immediate period just prior to the administration of the anaesthetic and when the child and parent are separated (Ellerton and Merriam, 1994). Carney *et al*'s (2003) study of children's views relating to hospitalisation identified many positive elements of the experience, such as the children feeling well-informed and the friendliness and helpfulness of staff. Negative perceptions related to the physical environment, such as the type of food and unsuitable play/recreational activities. Overwhelmingly, the provision of age-appropriate information was a vital component in promoting a positive experience (Carney *et al*, 2003).

Preparing the child and family for surgery and the general hospital experience is a vital component of pre-operative care and should begin during the first clinic appointment. Pre-operative preparation programmes are not a new phenomenon. Children of all ages express anxieties about pain, discomfort and being away from their family, and the lack of knowledge children have about hospitals necessitates the need for preparation programmes (Eiser and Patterson, 1984). As the child's age increases, needs shift from understanding the physical aspects of hospital to the social aspects of hospital, such as what is expected, visiting by friends, restrictions placed upon them, schooling, and the role of hospital staff (Eiser and Patterson, 1984). To be effective, preparation programmes need to ensure the content is appropriate to the child's needs (Price, 1991; Wynn, 1997). Pre-operative preparation strategies must meet the unique needs of the child, the cognitive ages of the children participating, and address the needs of the parents because their involvement is integral to the child's preparation (Carpenter, 1998; O'Conner-Von, 2000). Furthermore, it is vital that the preparation offered matches that desired by the child and family (Mitchell, 2000), and so it will be necessary to establish the level and depth of information each child and family wishes to receive. With the growing number of pre-operative preparation programmes, the effectiveness in terms of cost and direct benefits for the child and family between different types of programmes must be evaluated (O'Conner-Von, 2000).

Price (1991) undertook a comprehensive review of preparation programmes and concluded that, despite methodological weaknesses, these programmes have been shown to reduce anxiety for the child and family. Although the focus of the majority of the literature available is primarily a description of the preparation programmes, rather than an analysis of the benefits, the last decade has seen a steady increase in the amount of research relating to preparation of children for surgery (Ellerton and Merriam, 1994; O'Conner-Von, 2000). Furthermore, the quality of the research available, in terms of appropriate methodology, statistical testing and addressing issues of reliability and validity, appears to be improving (O'Conner-Von, 2000). There appears to be sufficient evidence to support the need for preparation programmes prior to surgery, which assist the child and family's ability to cope with the proposed surgery and post-operative care (O'Conner-Von, 2000). Many children's units have established programmes aimed at preparing children for hospitalisation. The variety of formats of these programmes include:

- Individual preparation, usually in the form of a visit to the surgical area at the time of the outpatient consultation, but could include preparation by telephone

- Group preparation, usually at a pre-arranged club or meeting, which often includes a tour of the facilities, play opportunities, and a question and answer session

- Group or individual play sessions

- Video recordings/slide show of the facilities and general procedures

- Written materials, such as information leaflets, colouring and storybooks.

With the increased used of information technology, the potential range of strategies for information provision is expanding and can include database links to local hospitals or national organisations (Mitchell, 2000). Ideally, the type of preparation programme must be appropriate for the individual child and family, and meet local needs (Carpenter, 1998; O'Conner-Von, 2000). It is inappropriate to expect families having lengthy distances to travel to attend a pre-admission preparation club, if it is held on a different day from the outpatient consultation (Acharya, 1992), while audio/visual tapes will only be appropriate for the child and family who speak the primary language in which the material is produced. Descriptions of the development of specific preparation programmes within the literature, include Gaughan and Sweeney's (1997) and Ellerton and Merriam's (1994) pre-admission day programmes, Stone and Glasper's (1997) information leaflets and Adams *et al*'s (1991) preparation booklet.

The child and family will require information relating to medical and anaesthetic equipment and techniques that will be encountered. The use of play can be an invaluable tool, which allows children to become familiar with and explore equipment in a safe and secure environment. The involvement of a play specialist during each of the perioperative stages can offer the child psychological support by allowing him/her to express his/her feelings (Webster, 2000). Play activities need to be appropriate to the child's age and capabilities.

Although pre-admission preparation can do much to alleviate the anxieties a child and family experience when coming into hospital, it should not replace the need to provide appropriate information and reassurance once the child is admitted. This should include allowing the child and family to express their concerns and anxieties and have their views and wishes respected and, wherever practically possible, included in the care delivered. The key principles healthcare professionals involved in the care of a child should consider when planning care, include:

- Every event in hospital has the potential to be frightening and evoke high levels of anxiety; there are no routine procedures for the child and family

- Preparation does not have to be elaborate, and information at the right level that is appropriate and sensitive can make a difference

- Involving parents in preparation requires them to have knowledge, be fully informed and feel valued and supported

- Parents and children do not necessarily ask for information; do not assume this is because they know everything; make the first move

- Finding out what knowledge already exists, including previous experiences, information from the media, and what the parents and child expect or perceive will happen

- Understanding age and stages of development, in order to appreciate differing perceptions, is vital

- Emergency admission is particularly stressful and may necessitate repeated explanations
- Effective communication is paramount
- Putting yourself in the position of child and family
- Revisiting your own working environment and practices.

(Taylor *et al*, 1999)

The development of preparation programmes appears to have become the domain of nursing, both ward and theatre staff, often aided by play specialists. There is much less literature available in relation to the role of parents in preparing their child for hospital, yet it is widely accepted that parents, with their intimate knowledge, are the best people for this role (Price, 1991; Stone and Glasper, 1997; Taylor *et al*, 1999). If parents are expected to take on this role, they require support and guidance, as well as knowledge about hospital procedures. Action for Sick Children provides a range of books and leaflets for parents, with information about preparing their child for hospital admission (*Appendix III*). In addition, parents may wish for advice relating to the timing of preparing for hospital. This will vary depending upon the age of the child. General preparation should begin in outpatients, ideally through the use of a play specialist, and may include an introduction to the ward and hospital environment. Older children should be included in discussions within the initial consultation, and facilitated to ask questions. It has been suggested young school-age children should be prepared during the week preceding surgery, allowing the child time to consider issues and ask questions (National Association of Welfare of Children in Hospital, 1987). For the younger child, who will have a limited concept of time, preparation one to two days prior to hospitalisation, with reinforcement on the day of admission, may be more beneficial (National Association of Welfare of Children in Hospital, 1987). The use of stories, colouring books and expression through play will greatly enhance a child's ability to explore ideas and feelings. Despite effective preparation, it cannot be overstressed that a young child's main concern will be the separation from parents and removal from the home environment, whereas an older child may be more concerned about process and procedures, and loss of control (Kain *et al*, 1996). Therefore preparing children for surgery and hospitalisation must include a major commitment to ensure practices and policies in relation to the overall philosophy of caring for the child and family are adhered to.

7.3 Day surgery

Ireland and Rushforth (1998a: 199) define day care as:

> '*the admission of children to hospital for all or part of a day, for the purpose of undergoing surgery, medical therapy, an investigative procedure or observation*'.

They suggest that the term 'day case' has been superceded by the term 'day care' to reflect the move away from day care units solely providing care for day case surgical children and to encompass the greater diversity of care provision. However, there is no doubt that surgeons were early advocates of day care, embracing its philosophy as early as the 1900s (Nicoll, 1909). Surgical day cases have often been the driving force behind the establishment of designated day care facilities for children, recognising the inability of acute inpatient wards to meet this group of children's needs adequately (Smith and Garner, 2001).

Advances in anaesthetics and anaesthesia techniques, the use of less invasive surgery (for example, laparoscopic and endoscopic techniques) and technological advances are resulting in the possible procedures suitable for day surgery reaching new heights. In fact, a recent report by the Paediatric Forum of the Royal College of Surgeons of England (2000) suggests that 75 percent of elective surgical procedures could be undertaken on a day basis for children. The actual number of day cases performed is probably much less than advocated. Data is collected in relation to inpatient and day care procedures within the National Health Service, but it is difficult to clearly identify the number of children who undergo day surgery. In part, this is due to the variability in the data collection, which is often specialty-based, differing interpretations of children in terms of age, and lack of inclusion of private hospital care. Many of the published reports relate to local data and often reflect service developments in favour of day care. Burn's (1983) review of day care in children indicated that only 40 percent of the total surgery conducted on children that could potentially be managed on a day care basis was undertaken as a day case. Various specialties were reviewed with only designated paediatric surgeons consistently using day care to its full potential. The data only represented the locality that formed the basis of the study, and information comparing regions, for example regional centres (where paediatric surgeons perform the majority of surgery on children) and smaller district general hospitals (where general surgeons perform the majority of surgery on children), is difficult to find. The increases in day care raises the question first posed by Ireland and Rushforth in 1998, namely: *Day care—in whose best interests?*

Day care has mutual advantages and disadvantages for the child and family, staff and service providers (*Table 7.3a*). The overwhelming advantage of providing day care facilities is to reduce inpatient hospitalisation for children, with its associated problems of acute distress, potential separation from family, psychological trauma and disruption to normal routines. Children admitted for minor surgery on a day basis demonstrated less behavioural changes and less disruption in nursery/school performance, within the three months after discharge, when compared with the children admitted for overnight stay as an inpatient group (Scaife and Campbell, 1988). In addition to reducing separation anxiety for the child and family, a further advantage for the child is the reduction of potentially frightening experiences and the number of healthcare professionals they will encounter (Ireland and Rushforth, 1998). However, the short duration of the admission may hinder the child and healthcare professionals developing a trusting relationship and often procedures can be rushed in the desire to ensure the child arrives in theatre on time, which may bewilder the child. Furthermore, anaesthetic techniques that may delay recovery, such as the use of a premedication and long-acting analgesia may be withheld, with the potential benefits of sedation and additional pain relief lost (Ireland and Rushforth, 1998).

Table 7.3a: Advantages and disadvantages of day care

Advantages	Disadvantages
Child ● Reduces psychological trauma ● Reduced exposure to stressful situations ● Reduced contact with different staff	*Child* ● May not be able to develop a relationship with staff ● Care may be rushed due to time frame ● Potential for increased period of fasting
Family ● Reduces stress for family, including easier to plan for one day, no risk of the admission being cancelled with associated disruptions ● Outline of day can be more specific ● Care can be more tailored to meet the child and family's needs	*Family* ● Increases burden of care for the family; may cause anxiety ● May require three hospital visits: outpatient, pre-admission clerking/assessment/and day treatment and a further visit for the child to become familiar with environment ● Educational information may be given all at once and be overwhelming ● May be difficult to access other members of multidisciplinary team on day of surgery, if additional input is required
Economic due to shorter hospital stay ● Staff salaries (no need to pay weekend and night enhancements) ● 'Hotel facilities' not needed ● Decreased risk of hospital-acquired infection	*Economic* ● May not be potentially viable for small units to have a separate children's day unit ● Cost transferred to primary healthcare setting
Service ● Improved recruitment of staff ● Improved planning of elective cases, which are not then competing for inpatient acute admissions ● Potential to reduce waiting lists	*Service* ● May be difficult for smaller hospitals to have separate unit, due to small numbers ● Delays in theatre if child is not prepared safely or arrives late
Staff ● More predictable working hours ● Part-time staff can contribute equally	*Staff* ● Fast throughput of children may not be rewarding ● Need to be alert to complications, promptly ● Need to recognise and act upon any child protection issues within a short time frame

Day care has enormous benefits for the family as a whole with less disruption to the family's routines, and the expense and commitments associated with visiting or staying with a child overnight. The family can plan better for time away from work, transport to and from hospital and arrangements for the childcare of siblings, which can be planned in advance. However, the burden of responsibility for the psychological and physical preparation of the child shifts from healthcare professionals to the parents (Ireland and Rushforth, 1998). Without appropriate resources and innovative working practices, this can leave families feeling isolated and ill prepared for this role (Dearmun, 1994). One particular area for concern is pre-operative fasting regimes (Ireland and Rushforth, 1998). Usual practice involves providing all the children with the same fasting time regardless of the position on the operating list, because the ordering of children is not usually done till much nearer the day of surgery, well after parents have been informed of the admission date (Neill, 1995). Solutions could include advanced planning of operating schedules with staggered admission times or telephone contact the day prior to admission for a specific fast time, both of which have resource implications. In addition to pre-operative preparation, parents must take on the responsibility for ongoing care following discharge (Ireland and Rushforth, 1998). This is an onerous responsibility and can be a daunting prospect for many families. James (1995) suggests the family should not feel pressured into day care treatment and, if they do not feel able to undertake the demands that will be placed upon them, be offered inpatient treatment. The child and family will required detailed discharge advice, both verbal and written, specific to the child's treatment and individual needs, appropriate discharge analgesia, telephone contacts and community nursing support (James, 1995).

In addition to the benefits of day care for the child and family, there are benefits for the services providers and staff. The most obvious benefits for service providers are economic, as a direct result of reduced staff salaries (no weekend and night enhancement costs) and not requiring 'hotel facilities'. Other less tangible benefits include the potential decreased risk of hospital-acquired infection and saving on recruitment due to increased retention of staff. In today's climate of meeting waiting list targets, designated day care units are attractive because it is very unlikely that children will be cancelled at short notice. Children admitted to a designated day care unit will not be competing for beds with inpatient acute admissions and there is potential to improve waiting lists due to increased throughput of children. Staff working in designated day units will have more predictable working hours. Disadvantages include the fast throughput of children may result in the caring aspect of nursing children being less rewarding, and that day care is often negatively perceived, by the unenlightened, as a less technical area of child care provision (Thornes, 1991; Wigens, 1997). Staff employed to work in day care units should be selected on their motivation, enthusiasm and commitment to day care provision, not purely on their desire for more predictable working hours (James, 1995). Within nursing, the potential for nurses within day care to lead and develop services has not yet been realised (Smith and Garner, 2001). The development of advanced nurse practitioners' roles within the ambulatory care setting has the potential to have a massive impact upon child health nursing (Dearmun and Gordon, 1999).

Many of the advantages of day care that have been outlined will only be realised if the service provision is appropriate to meet the needs of the child undergoing day care, and selection criteria are appropriate. Patient selection must begin in the outpatient department and needs to consider the suitability of the procedure for day care, anaesthetic risk, and parents' abilities and commitment to day care. Other practical considerations include parents' access to a telephone and suitable transport home. The Royal College of Surgeons (1992) has suggested that operations suitable for day care should be relatively easy to perform and of a short duration (less than one hour), with minimal potential post-operative complications or disruption to normal functioning, and not requiring complex analgesia regimes. The risk of anaesthesia is an important consideration and only those children falling into low risk categories should be offered treatment on a day basis. The American Society of Anaesthesiologists (Mak *et al*, 2002) classified physical status in relation to anaesthesia risk, and grades low risk patients as:

- Normal health individuals
- Mild systemic disease that is well controlled and does not cause functional limitations.

Infants under 46 weeks of gestation or less than 5 kilos in weight are usually considered unsuitable for day care because the risk of anaesthetic apnoea significantly increases in this age group (Welborn *et al*, 1986). Day care units should have clear admission criteria to ensure that children are suitable for day care.

Day care should not compromise the outcome of the treatment. Current evidence suggests that in relation to managing post-operative nausea and vomiting, urine retention (following circumcision) and wound infection, there are no differences between day care and inpatient groups (Scaife and Campbell, 1988). Nausea and vomiting and urine retention did result in a number (8 percent) of day care children requiring overnight admission. Community nurses managed wound problems effectively.

It is more than a decade since the publication of *Just for the Day* (Thornes, 1991), which contained the first comprehensive principles for the care of children admitted for the day within the UK. *Just for the Day* represented several disciplines (Royal College of Nursing, British Paediatric Association, National Association of Health Authorities and Trusts and National Association of Welfare of Children Hospital) and aimed to recommend good practice for children requiring day care, in light of the enormous variation in quality and service provision. Although the report describes a range of models for the provision of day care, it clearly recommends the best option is a designated *'children's day unit admitting both medical and surgical patients'* (p21). Where this is not a viable proposition, other possibilities include:

- A day area situated in a children's ward used solely for the admission of day children (both medical and surgical)

- A day room used solely for children admitted for medical investigations

- Dedicated sessions within an adult day unit, used solely for the treatment of children requiring surgery. Children are not nursed alongside adult patients and the environment is easily converted into a child-friendly area.

The report recommended that whichever system of care delivery is adopted, the 12 quality standards for the day care of children should be achievable. These twelve standards have become the benchmarks for paediatric day care:

1. The admission is planned in an integrated way to include pre-admission, day of admission and post-admission care, and to incorporate the concept of a planned transfer of care to primary and/or community services

2. The child and parent are offered preparation both before and during the day of admission

3. Specific written information is provided to ensure that parents understand their responsibilities throughout the episode

4. The child is admitted to an area designated for day cases and not mixed with acutely ill patients

5. The child is neither admitted nor treated alongside adults

6. The child is cared for by identified staff specifically designated to the day care area

7. Medical, nursing and all other staff are trained for, and skilled in, working with children and their families, in addition to the expertise needed for day case work

8. The organisation and delivery of care are planned specifically for day cases so that every child is likely to be discharged within the day

9. The building, equipment and furnishings comply with safety standards for children

10. The environment is homely and includes areas for play and other activities designed for children and young people

11. Essential documentation, including communication with the primary and/or community services, is completed before each child goes home so that after-care and follow-up consultations are not delayed

12. Once care has been transferred to the home, nursing support is provided by nurses trained in the care of sick children

(Thornes, 1991: 6)

The principles within *Just for the Day* (Thornes, 1991) can be used as a framework for the establishment of a day care unit and the development of specific policies relating to children requiring day care (Smith and Garner, 2001). This ensures the care delivered is driven by the needs of the children and not the needs of the service. Where possible, day care should be an integral part of the children's services, and thus benefits from having access to the wider team (nutritional nurses, continence adviser, pain service) and makes particularly effective use of the children's outreach service. Maintaining links with other children's areas is essential, preventing practice from developing in isolation or becoming outdated and stagnating. Unfortunately, many service providers do not have sufficient numbers of children to develop separate day care facilities, which would be under utilised and a drain on resources, and there is difficulty in recruiting children's nurses when the sole commitment is not nursing children (Solly, 2001). Practical solutions include:

- Career incentives that offer higher grades to children' nurses working in adult day areas, which reflects the expectations that they will contribute to developments of the services and make appropriate links with colleagues in children's services

- A lead nurse responsible for the standards of care for the children on the day unit

- Supporting the children's nurse within adult units by rotating nursing and play specialist staff from children's areas; these staff should have an interest in day care

- Adult colleagues working in areas where children are nursed should have, as part of their in-service, educational input into the needs of the child and basic paediatric life-support training.

(Solly, 2001)

It is over a decade since the publication of *Just for the Day* (Thornes, 1991) and, although inappropriate to suggest that all of the principles of the report have been achieved nationally, there is enormous potential for developing children's day services.

Children's nurse practitioners are a growing phenomenon within the UK (Truobranski, 1994). Studies from the United States have demonstrated how these nurses are able to assess patients, have knowledge of both the overview and intimate details of the planned care, and are effective in collaboration with other professionals (Kirkpatrick, 1994). Although there are a number of initiatives developing the role of the neonatal nurse practitioner, the nurse practitioner movement within general children's nursing is not well developed (Dearmun and Gordon, 1999). There appears to be an uncomfortable transition period where nurses are undertaking extended roles, such as cannulation and venepuncture, requesting X-rays and prescribing medication on one hand, but are questioning the role of these new tasks within a framework for providing holistic care (Dearmun and Gordon, 1999; Silver and McAteep, 1988). Nurses with suitable training are capable of developing many of the routine tasks that have previously been in the domain of the junior doctor. If this is linked to a framework of providing holistic care to the child and family, with improvements in service provision, these initiatives should be developed. It is highly conceivable that nurse-led children's day care units are a realistic way forward, as nurses working in children's day care are able to provide seamless care, with minimal disruption to the child and family's normal daily lives by putting the child and family foremost. Many areas of care are already within the remit of nursing responsibilities in day care, such as venepuncture and cannulation, and nurse discharging (Smith and Garner, 2001). Others areas of care which could potentially be managed by the nursing team include drug prescribing, particularly post-operative analgesia (which could be incorporated into existing pain management guidelines) and pre-operative clerking by nursing staff. These developments could potentially improve the quality of care, which at times can be rushed and even delay theatre start times when junior doctors may be dealing with inpatient children. There is no doubt that, with resources to provide additional education and support for the nursing staff, there is tremendous scope for nurse-led day care units.

7.4 Continuing care in the community

Bia (1998) suggests that the increasing complexity of children's needs, advances in technology and government directives have resulted in the expansion of secondary community-based services for children. In addition, major societal changes, such as reduction of support from extended family due to increased mobilisation, increased poverty, increased homelessness, increased single families and a more diverse culture, have the potential to influence the type and function of service provisions. The advantages of developing care in the community (Bradley, 1997; Eaton, 2000; Jester and Turner, 1998; National Health Service Executive, 1996) include:

- Facilitates early discharge

- The potential to minimise the psychological sequelae of lengthy hospitalisation by reducing the number of nights children require to be in hospital

- Maximises growth and development

- A reduction in hospital-acquired infections

- Reduces travelling for the child and family

- Promotes family life and functioning

- The potential to assist in the blurring of boundaries between health, social and educational services, which is particularly pertinent for children with complex and special needs

- Improved collaboration between primary and secondary care

- Facilitates closer therapeutic relationships due to child and family having greater contact with a smaller healthcare team

- The provision of services that reflect the wishes of the child and family.

The disadvantages of community-based service provision (Jester and Turner, 1998) include:

- Increased costs for primary care service providers without transfer of funds from secondary care services

- The lack of immediate access to the full range of healthcare professionals' equipment and investigations

- Lack of respite care

- A high degree of responsibility is transferred from healthcare professionals to the family

- Lack of privacy at home due to visits from healthcare professionals

- Lack of sleep for the main carer, which is influenced by the dependency and care needs of the child

- Increased stress for the family and the main carer, particularly if the child requires constant supervision

- Equipment can often be bulky and noisy

- Financial difficulties, particularly if one member of the family has to give up or reduce working hours

- Disruption to the family's normal routines.

The House of Commons Select Committee (1997) recommended that all children requiring nursing care within the community should have access and be cared for by an appropriately qualified children's nurse. Service provision should be available 24 hours a day and every general practitioner should be able to refer a child to a community children's nurse for care if needed. However, these recommendations are far from being realised due to funding difficulties and inadequate numbers of community children's nurses. The inequalities include variations in service provision, depending upon geographical location, and many families being denied access to specific children's services (Eaton, 2000; Smith, 2000). The British Paediatric Association (BPA, 1993) predicted a growth of secondary acute care outside the hospital domain, and there are now over 250 community children's nursing teams within the United Kingdom (Royal College of Nursing, 2000). Despite the increasing number of community children's nursing teams, they have developed in an *ad hoc* manner without a national strategic direction.

Community care provision for children has, in general, developed in response to local need and circumstances, rather than based upon any rational analysis of healthcare needs, in terms of both the most effective type of service or cost considerations (Royal College of Nursing, 2000; Smith, 2000). The various models for providing community children's nursing include: the nurse delivering specialised care (usually linked to a regional centre) or generalist services, the service based in either the community or the hospital, and the funding of services either from community trusts, acute trusts or charities (Royal College of Nursing, 2000). Eaton's (2000) review of children's community nursing services identified six models of service provision that have developed within the United Kingdom. *Table 7.4a* outlines these models and their relative advantages and disadvantages.

Table 7.4a: Models of community children's nursing services, and their relative advantages and disadvantages (adapted from Bradley, 1997; Eaton, 2000; Jester and Turner, 1998)

Model	Characteristics	Advantages	Disadvantages
Hospital outreach: generalist	The team is based in the hospital. Care is usually provided by generalist children's nurses.	Easier for staff to build up a relationship with the discharging team and the family prior to discharge. May be able to provide access to nursing staff 24 hours a day, 7 days a week.	May be more difficult to liaise and develop effective working relationships with the range of community healthcare professionals. Staff may have dual responsibilities between inpatients and children nursed in the community.
Hospital outreach: specialist	Care is generally administered by hospital staff and usually to a specific client group. Care is provided by specialist children's nurses.	Easier for staff to build up a relationship with the discharging team and the family prior to discharge. Often involved in the specialist care delivered in hospital and the education of parents prior to discharge. May be able to provide cover 24 hours per day, 7 days a week, but this may not necessarily be specialist services.	May be more difficult to liaise and develop effective working relationships with the range of community healthcare professionals. Staff may have dual responsibilities between inpatients and children nursed in the community.
Community-based children' nursing teams	The team is based in the community which supplies services to a defined geographical area. Care provided by children's nurses specifically trained in community care.	Sole commitment to children nursed in the community. Knowledge of the range of community services available and can build up effective relationships with other community-based staff.	Children's nurses may be working in isolation Poor communication between hospital and community. Less access to specialised equipment.

Model	Characteristics	Advantages	Disadvantages
Hospital at home	The team can be based either in hospital or community and carries out complex treatments in the home. Care is given by qualified child health nurses, usually with additional specialist knowledge.	Often allows high dependency children to be nursed at home. Easier for staff to build up a relationship with the discharging team and family prior to discharge. Often involved in the specialist care delivered in hospital and education of parents prior to discharge. May be able to provide cover 24 hours per day, 7 days a week, but this may not necessarily be specialist services.	May be more difficult to liaise and develop effective working relationships with the range of community healthcare professionals. Staff may have dual responsibilities between inpatients and children nursed in the community.
District nursing services	Adult-based community nursing scheme. Staff have community training but not necessarily child health training.	Sole commitment to patients nursed in the community. Knowledgeable in the range of community services available and can build up effective relationships with other community-based staff. May be able to provide cover 24 hours per day, 7 days a week.	May lack theoretical knowledge relating to child health issues. May not be able to build up expertise in caring for children. Adult workload may take priority. Poor communication between hospital and community. Less access to specialised equipment.
Ambulatory or assessment unit	Diverse range of service provision usually delivered in community practice or day care facility within a hospital. Care given by range of staff who may have a child health qualification.	Staff experienced in ambulatory care provision.	Often services restricted to the opening hours of the unit. May lack theoretical knowledge of child health issues. May not be able to build up expertise in caring for children. Adult workload may take priority. Access may be restricted to unit opening times.

Healthcare professionals responsible for children receiving community care need to be knowledgeable in both child health and community issues (Eaton, 2001). However, most services, although working towards this goal, have been established without being able to recruit dual-qualified staff. Eaton (2001) suggests tension exists between the models of service provision, such as the skills offered, defining boundaries, threatened existing roles, and working practices. These differences need to be put aside in order to ascertain the most effective type of service provision for children nursed in the community, in terms of quality of service provision and cost effectiveness. In the present era of evidence-based practice and escalating healthcare costs, there needs to be a detailed evaluation of these services in respect of outcomes compared with hospital-based care, such as medical complications, re-admission rates, infection rates, child and parent satisfaction and cost-benefit analysis (Bradley, 1997; Eaton, 2000).

Parents, although positive about early discharge, have many apprehensions about their ability to provide ongoing care for their child (Thornes, 1991). In the absence of specific community services, parents experience difficulties following discharge and these include:

- The discharge procedure; many parents did not feel prepared to care for their child following discharge and were unable to express their concerns, accepting the discharge date as inevitable

- Lack of information; often information (verbal and written) was not explained and parents' understanding was not checked

- Parents felt isolated and anxious

- Parents felt they needed reassurance; this type of support was often not available

- Specific advice in relation to their child's needs was not available

- Continuity of care was absent; many parents were not given a contact point; those that were felt that advice given was not consistent and contacts did not have any knowledge about their child's needs.

(Smith, 2000)

Where services to support children in the community exist, parents 'without exception' appear deeply satisfied with the support provided (Burr, 1998: 14). This satisfaction is understandable if the aims of providing community care, that are to prevent or minimise hospitalisation, maximise growth and development, promote family independence and normal family functioning, are achieved (Bradley, 1997). The reviews of service developments (Bradley, 1997; Eaton, 2000) suggest that services have been developed to meet a wide range of children's needs—chronic and life-threatening illness, complex care needs, facilitating the early discharge of children with acute illnesses requiring medical treatment—and to support the reduction of stay for planned surgical admissions. It would appear that the majority of services reviewed are aimed at the child with ongoing complex healthcare needs. This potentially leaves many children who have undergone minor surgery without adequate provision. In addition, the range of surgical specialties may contribute to an inability, due to the small numbers of children, to allow the development of community services to meet these children's needs. Funding specialised services, which are expensive, can be problematic (Hennessy, 1994).

Hogg's (1994) standards for children undergoing surgery stresses that, following surgery, consideration should be given to specific areas of care, such as eating and drinking, pain management, mobilisation and wound management. In addition, with the increasingly shortened hospital stay, these areas of care require ongoing support once the child is discharged. Furthermore, many children with complex needs may require repeated surgery and specialised nursing care. Both groups of children and their families require and deserve the support of child health community services, and care delivered by staff educated and skilled in meeting their specific needs.

References

Acharya S (1992) Assessing the need for pre-admission visit. *Paediatr Nurs* 9(4): 20–23

Adams J, Gill S, McDonald M (1991) Reducing Fear in Hospital. *Nurs Times* 87(1): 62–64

Ainsworth MDS, Blehar MC, Waters E, Wall S (1978) *Patterns of Attachment: A Psychological Study of the Strange Situation.* Lawrence Erlbaum Associates, Hillsdale

Alsop-Shields L, Mohay H (2001) John Bowlby and James Robertson: theorists, scientists and crusaders for improvements in the care of children in hospital. *J Adv Nurs* 35(1): 50–58

Audit Commission (1993) *Children First: A Study of Hospital Services.* HMSO, London

Bar-Haim Y, Sutton S, Fox A *et al* (2000) Stability and change of attachment at 14, 24, and 58 months of age: behavior, representation, and life events. *J Child Psychol Psychiatry* 42(3): 381–88

Bia RE (1998) Community outreach for children with complex needs. In: Glasper EA, Lowson S eds. *Innovations in Paediatric Ambulatory Care: A Nursing Perspective.* Macmillan Press, London

Bowlby J (1979) *The Making and Breaking of Affectional Bonds.* Tavistock Publications, London

Bowlby J (1951) *Maternal Care and Mental Health.* World Health Organization, Geneva

Bradley (1997) Better late than never? An evaluation of community nursing services for children in the UK. *J Clin Nurs* 32(1): 49–56

Bridger P, Rees M (1995) What a difference a day makes. *Health Serv J* 105: 22–23.

British Paediatric Association (1993) *Flexible Options for Paediatric Care: A Discussion Document.* BPA, London

Burn JMB (1983) Responsible use of resources in day surgery. *Br Med J* 286: 492–93

Burr S (1998) Home comforts. *Nurs Stand* 12(27): 14

Carney T, Murphy S, McClure J *et al* (2003) Children's views of hospitalization: an exploratory study of data collection. *J Child Health Care* 7(1): 27–39

Carpenter KH (1998) Developing a pediatric/parent hospital preparation program. *AORN J* 67(5): 1042–46

Clarke AM, Clarke ADB (1976) *Early Experience: Myth and Evidence.* Open Books, London

Crocker E (1980) Reactions of children to healthcare encounters. In: Robinson GC, Clark HF, eds. *The Hospital Care of Children; A Review of Contemporary Issues*. University Press, New York

Dearmun AK (1994) Defining differences: children's day surgery. *Surgical Nurse* 7(6): 7–11

Dearmun A K, Gordon K (1999) The nurse practitioner in children's ambulatory care. *Paediatr Nurs* 11(1): 18–21

Department of Health (1991) *Welfare of Children and Young People in Hospital*. HMSO, London

Douglas JWB (1975) Early hospital admission and later behaviour and learning. *Devel Med Child Neurol* 17: 456–48

Draijer N, Langland W (1999) Childhood trauma and perceived parental dysfunction in the etiology of dissociative symptoms in psychiatric inpatients. *Am J Psychiatry* 156(3): 379–85

Eaton N (2000) Children's community nursing services; models of care delivery. A review of the United Kingdom literature. *J Adv Nurs* 32(1): 49–56

Eiser C, Patterson D (1984) Children's perceptions of hospital: a preliminary study. *Int J Nurs Stud* 21: 45–50

Ellerton ML, Merriam C (1994) Preparing children and families psychologically for day surgery: an evaluation. *J Adv Nurs* 19(6): 1057–62

Gaughan M, Sweeney E (1997) Take heart: setting up a pre-admission day. *Paediatr Nurs* 9(1): 22–23

Glasper EA, Lowson S (1998) *Innovations in Paediatric Ambulatory Care: A Nursing Perspective*. Macmillan Press, London

Goodman S, Adams C (1989) 'Uncumphtable'. *Nurs Times* 85(49) 28–31

Hawthorn P (1974) *Nurse I Want My Mummy!* Royal College of Nursing, London

Hennessy D (1993) Purchasing community nursing care. *Paediatr Nurs* 5(2): 10–12

Hogg C (1994) *Setting Standards for Children Undergoing Surgery*. Action for Sick Children, London

House of Commons Health Select Committee (1997) *Health Services for Children and Young People in the Community, Home and School: Fifth Report*. Stationery Office, London

Ireland L, Rushforth H (1998) Day care—in whose best interests? *Paediatr Nurs* 10(5): 15–19

Ireland I, Rushforth H (1998a) Paediatric day care and its contribution to ambulatory care nursing. In: Glasper EA, Lowson S, eds. *Innovations in Paediatric Ambulatory Care: A Nursing Perspective*. Macmillan Press, London

James J (1995) Day care admissions. *Paediatr Nurs* 7(1): 25–37

Jester R, Turner D (1998) Hospital at home: the Bromsgrove experience. *Nurs Stand* 12(20): 40–42

Kain ZN, Mayes LC, O'Connor TZ *et al* (1996) Preoperative anxiety in children: predictors and outcomes. *Arch Pediatric Adolesc Med* 150(12): 1238–45

Kirkpartick S (1994) Nurse practitioners step in to keep pace with growing day surgery. *Assoc Operat Room Nurses* 40(65): 826–27

LaMontagne LL, Hepworth JT, Johnson BD *et al* (1996) Children's preoperative coping and its effects on postoperative anxiety and return to normal activity. *Nurs Res* 45(3): 141–47

Mak PHK, Campbell RCH, Irwin MG (2002) The ASA physical status classification: inter-observer consistency. *Anaesthet Intens Care* 30: 633–40

Ministry of Health (1959) *The Welfare of Children in Hospital: Report of the Committee on the Welfare of Children in Hospital (Platt Report)*. HMSO, London

Ministry of Health (1946) *Report of the Care of Children Committee (Curtis Report)*. HMSO, London

Miron J (1990) What children think about hospitals. *Can Nurse* 86(3): 23–25

Mitchell M (2000) Nursing intervention for pre-operative anxiety. *Nurs Stand* 14(3): 40–43

National Association of Welfare of Children in Hospital (1987) *Emotional Needs of Children Undergoing Surgery*. NAWCH, London

National Health Service Executive (1996) *Child Health in the Community: A Guide to Good Practice*. Department of Health, London

Neill S (1995) Fasting for day surgery: parental role. *Paediatr Nurs* 7(2): 20–23

Nicoll J (1909) The surgery of infancy. *Br Med J* 2: 753–54

O'Conner-Von S (2000) Preparing children for surgery—an integrative research review. *AORN J* 71(2): 334–43

Paediatric Forum of the Royal College of Surgeons (2000) *Children's Surgery—A First Class Service*. Royal College of Surgeons, London

Price B (1988) What are nurses like? *Nurs Times* 84(1): 42–43

Price S (1991) Preparing children for admission to hospital. *Nurs Times* 27(9): 46–49

Robertson J (1970) *Young Children in Hospital,* 2nd edn. Tavistock Publications Limited, London

Robertson J (1958) *Going to Hospital with Mother (film).* Tavistock Institute of Human Relations, London

Robertson J (1955) Young children in long-term hospitals. *Nurs Times* **23**: 63–65

Rodin J (1983) *Will This Hurt?* Royal College of Nursing, London

Royal College of Nursing (2000) *Children's Community Nursing: Promoting Effective Teamworking for Children and their Families.* Royal College of Nursing, London

Royal College of Surgeons of England (1992) *Guidelines for Day Surgery.* Royal College of Surgeons, London

Rutter M (1981) *Maternal Deprivation Reassessed,* 2nd edn. Penguin, Harmondsworth

Rutter M (1972) *Maternal Deprivation Reassessed.* Penguin, Harmondsworth

Scaife JM, Campbell I (1988) A comparison of the outcome of day care and in-patient treatment of paediatric surgical cases. *J Child Psychol Psychiatry* **29**(2): 185–98

Schaffer HR, Emerson PE (1964) The development of social attachments in children. *Monographs of Social Research in Child Development* **29**(3)

Shaffer DR (2002) *Developmental Psychology, Childhood and Adolescence,* 5th edn. Brooks/Coles Publishing, USA

Sheldon L (1997) Hospitalising children: a review of the effects. *Nurs Stand* **12**(1): 44–47

Shirley PJ, Thompson N, Kenward M *et al* (1998) Parental anxiety before elective surgery in children: a British perspective. *Anaesthesia* **53**(10): 956–59

Silver H K, McAteep PI (1988) Should nurses be substitute house officers? *Am J Nurs* **12**: 1671–73

Smith J, Garner T (2001) Focus on children's day care—past, present and future. *J One Day Surg* **10**(4): 10–11

Smith L (2000) Weaving the seamless web of care: an analysis of parents' perceptions of their needs following discharge of their child from hospital. *J Adv Nurs* **31**(4): 812–20

Solly J (2001) Commentary on: focus on children's day care—past, present and future. *J One Day Surg* **10**(4): 11–12

Stone KJ H, Glasper EA (1997) Can leaflets assist parents in preparing children for hospital? *Br J Nurs* **6**(18): 1054–58

Taylor J, Müller DJ, Wattley L, Harris P (1999) *Nursing Children, Psychology Research and Practice*, 3rd edn. Stanley Thornes, Cheltenham

Teichman Y, Rafael MB, Lerman M (1986) Anxiety reaction of hospitalized children. *Br J Medic Psychol* 59: 375–82

Thomas A, Chess S (1977) *Temperament and Development*. Brunner/Mazel, New York

Thornes R (1991) *Just for the Day*. NAWCH, London

Truobranski PH (1994) Nurse practitioner: redefining the role of the community nurse. *J Adv Nurs* 19(1): 134

Turner G (1998) Parents' experiences of ambulatory care. *Paediatr Nurs* 10(8): 12–16

Vernon DTA, Foley JM, Sipowicz RR *et al* (1965) *The Psychological Responses of Children to Hospitalization and Illness*. Charles C Thomas, Springfield

Visintainer MA, Wolfer JA (1975) Psychological preparation for surgical patients: the effect on children's and parents' stress responses and adjustment. *Pediatrics* 56: 187–202

Waters E, Merrick S, Treboux *et al* (2000) Attachment security in infancy and early adulthood: a twenty-year longitudinal study. *Child Devel* 71(3) 684–89

Webster A (2000) The facilitating role of the play specialist. *Paediatr Nurs* 12(7): 24–27

Welborn LG, Ramirez N, Oh TH *et al* (1986) Post-anesthetic apnea and period breathing in infants. *Anesthesiol* 65: 658–61

Wigens L (1997) The conflict between 'new nursing' and 'scientific management' as perceived by surgical nurses. *J Adv Nurs* 25: 1116–22

Wynn B (1997) Pre-operative psychological preparation in pre-school age children: differences between research and practice. *Aus Paediatr Nurse* 6(1): 45–48

SUMMARY OF PIAGET'S (1953) STAGES OF COGNITIVE DEVELOPMENT

Sensori-motor stage (0-2 years)	Babies begin to discover the relationship between what they do and the consequence. They learn through the senses and physical activities. Infants begin to coordinate sensory inputs and motor capabilities; they develop from responding in a relatively reflex manner to developing complex sensorimotor co-ordinations and some problem-solving skills. Infants begin to develop a mental schema of an object or event and use this, as a basis for comparison, when faced with a new experience. Babies and infants need the opportunity to explore their surroundings and new objects. There begins a recognition of self and others; toddlers may be able to point to some external body parts. Illness is only an issue unless it interferes with their comfort and attachment with family. Treatments and procedures will only be understood in terms of what it is that happens and how it affects them, particularly personal comfort. Psychological consequences of stress may include withdrawal from surroundings, nightmares and being uncooperative.
Pre-operational stage (2-7 years)	Children in this age group are egocentric, do not understand there may be a different view from their own. They respond to objects and events in the way things appear to them. Objects may be invested with life and are often be used symbolically. They cannot distinguish between cause and effect. Pre-school children may be able to point to external body parts and have some understanding of their relationships but will not be able to make links with illness. School children begin to develop some understanding of illness and its effects upon desired activities. In this age group the child may believe someone is responsible for the pain and may view it as a punishment, which if they 'behave' will magically go away. Illness is often related to things happening to them and attributed to external concrete phenomena. There is comprehension of medicine but it is often in terms of magical happenings and there is over generalization. They may find specific tasks (such as injections, wearing safety helmet) difficult to understand, because they do not seem relevant to the present.

Concrete operational (7-12 years)	Children understand the basic properties of objects and their relationship with everyday events. They begin to acquire the mental components of logical thought and can understand complex tasks; meanings are often be taken literally. They develop some rational thinking: 'if' and 'when' situation. Late school children begin to understand complexities of anatomy and physiology, with some understanding of internal and external body parts and their function but these might be global, undifferentiated and laced with fantasy, each organ viewed in isolation. Can understand illness in terms of contamination or physical contacts. School children are intrigued by procedures and often pleased to help. Pain is physical and can be related to body parts; fear of harm may be strong.
Formal operational (12 years and older)	The major change within this age group is the depth to understanding, development of logical thinking, which is no longer confined to the concrete or observable. Can engage in pondering and hypothesis and imagine alternatives to events and offer many solutions to a problem. However, they may not be consistent in their thinking. They often imagine sinister consequences of any illness.

Piaget J (1952) *The Origins of Intelligence in Children.*
International University Press, New York

SUMMARY OF ERIKSON'S (1963) DEVELOPMENT CYCLE: THE EIGHT AGES OF MAN

Stage I **Trust vs. mistrust** (first year of life)	A sense of trust develops through the infant feeling physical comfort and by ensuring basic needs such as feeding are met. Trust developed in infancy sets the stage for a life-long expectation that the world will be a good and pleasant place in which to live. A tentative link is made between the support parents provide an infant in developing trust with an ability to foster spiritual well-being. This stage of development is a prototype for the future; trust developed in infancy provides a foundation for positive life expectations, and an absence of basic trust can present in later life with difficulties forming relationships.
Stage II **Autonomy vs. shame and doubt** (late infancy and toddler hood)	After gaining trust in the caregivers, infants discover that their behaviour is their own and begin to assert their sense of independence or autonomy; they realise their will. If restrained too hard they develop a sense of shame and doubt. Certainly this is a time when children are fascinated with magic and mystery, and may express themselves in fantasy and elaborate thoughts.
Stage III **Initiative vs. guilt** (pre-school years)	The child experiences a challenging, widening social world where active, purposeful behaviour is needed to cope with these challenges. Children begin to assume responsibility for their bodies, their behaviour, their toys and their pets. Developing a sense of responsibility increases initiative. Uncomfortable guilt feelings may arise if the child is irresponsible and then made to feel too anxious. However, guilt is compensated for by a feeling of achievement.
Stage IV **Industry vs. inferiority** (junior school years)	Children's initiative brings them into contact with a wealth of new experiences. As they move into middle and late childhood, they direct their energy towards mastering knowledge and intellectual skills. At no other time is the child more enthusiastic about learning than at the end of this period of expansive imagination; children like stories and narratives. If suppressed there is a danger of the child feeling inferior, unproductive and incompetent. This natural need for knowledge can be fostered and developed.
Stage V **Identity vs. identity confusion** (adolescence)	Individuals attempt to find out who they are and where they are going. Adolescents are faced with many new roles, for example social, relationships and vocational, which they need to explore in a healthy manner and should be neither pushed nor restricted; confusion over their own identity may occur.
Stage VI **Intimacy vs. isolation** (early adult)	Individuals attempt to form intimate relationships with others, i.e. finding oneself yet losing oneself to another.

Stage VII **Generativity vs. stagnation** (middle adulthood)	Generativity occurs through assisting the younger generation in developing and leading useful lives, whereas stagnation may occur if there appears to be no purpose to activities.
Stage VIII **Integrity vs. despair** (late adulthood)	A time of looking back and evaluating what we have done with our lives. Through many different routes the older person may have developed a positive outlook in most or all of the previous stages of development; if so, the retrospective glances will reveal a life well spent and a feeling of satisfaction.

Erikson E H (1963) *Childhood and Society*. 2nd edition.
WW Norton and Company, New York.

RESOURCES SUPPORTING PARENTS TO PREPARE CHILDREN FOR HOSPITAL

There is a wealth of resources to assist parents in preparing children for hospital. Many are available from Action for Sick Children and include:

Information leaflets for example

- Helping children cope with pain
- Going to outpatients
- Helping children to cope with needles
- Teenagers in hospital
- Herbies Heroes

Parents pack designed to help parents prepare their child for hospital which includes activities, puzzles, crayons and balloons for children.

Videos for example

- A visit to children's outpatients
- Jane's operation
- Coping with hospital

Action for Sick Children, C/o National Children's Bureau, 8 Wakley Street, London, EC1V 7OE
www.actionforsickchildren.org

KEY FACTORS

Key factors that should be considered when formulating local guidelines relating to the management and care of children with a morphine infusion

Key Factor		Associated considerations
Pain management strategy	1	Is there a need to change current attitudes towards pain?
	2	Is there an overall strategy for managing pain which includes complex analgesia systems?
	3	Is there a pain team with designated staff to address issues at local level?
	4	Are roles and responsibilities clearly outlined?
	5	Will there be group directives?
	6	Are pain assessment tools in use?
	7	Are criteria available to determine suitability of child?
	8	Is there a strategy/guideline for the implementation of continuous/patient/nurse controlled analgesia or a combination to be implemented?
	9	If patient/nurse controlled analgesia is an option, will there be a concurrent background infusion?
	10	What strategies are available if pain is not being managed effectively?
	11	Is a pain algorithm available?
	12	How, who and when will quality issues such as audit, service evaluations, and child and family satisfaction, be undertaken?
	13	How will critical incidents be reported and managed?
	14	How and who will review the guidelines?
Drug formulations	1	Are there protocols for standard infusion drug preparations?
	2	Will infusions be prepared on the ward or in pharmacy?
	3	Are there protocols for recommended drug dosages and infusion rates?
	4	Who will take responsibility for prescribing analgesia?
	5	What adjuvant drugs will be prescribed?

Key Factor		Associated considerations
Equipment (infusion pumps)	I	Is there sufficient and appropriate equipment, such as 'high risk' lockable pumps?
	2	Is equipment standardised throughout the trust?
	3	Have medical physics been involved with identifying, checking and maintaining equipment?
	4	How will equipment malfunctions be managed?
Equipment (consumables)	I	Are appropriate consumables available e.g. 50ml leur lock syringes, non-returnable valve, type of tubing, labels for lines?
Care of the child	I	Are there clear guidelines as to where the child will be nursed post-operatively?
	2	Are there adequate information leaflets for the child and family?
	3	Does the care system support child and family involvement?
	4	Is there a detailed care plan relating to pain management?
	5	Is there appropriate documentation?
	6	What type of monitoring and frequency of observations will be required?
	7	Are current observation charts satisfactory? Can pain and sedation scores be recorded?
	8	How will side-effects such as respiratory depression, urinary retention, erythema and itch, nausea and vomiting be managed?
	9	Are trouble-shooting guidelines available?
Education	I	Will there be multidisciplinary education and how will this be achieved?
	2	How will staff demonstrate competencies in care of morphine infusions?
	3	Who will assess staff and review effectiveness of educational packages?

Key factors that should be considered when formulating local guidelines relating to the management and care of children with an epidural infusion

Key Factor		Associated considerations
Pain management	1	Is there a need to change current attitudes towards pain?
	2	Is there an overall strategy for managing pain which includes complex analgesia systems?
	3	Is there a pain team with designated staff to address issues at local level?
	4	Are roles and responsibilities clearly outlined?
	5	Will there be group directives?
	6	Are pain assessment tools in use?
	7	Are criteria available to determine suitability of child?
	8	What strategies are available if pain is not being managed effectively?
	9	Is a pain algorithm available?
	10	How, who and when will quality issues such as audit, service evaluations, and child and family satisfaction, be undertaken?
	11	How will critical incidents be reported and managed?
	12	How and who will review the guidelines strategy
Drug formulations	1	Are there protocols for standard infusion drug preparations?
	2	Will infusions be prepared on the ward or in pharmacy?
	3	Are there protocols for recommended drug dosages and infusion rates?
	4	Who will take responsibility for prescribing analgesia?
	5	What adjuvant drugs will be prescribed?
Equipment (infusion pumps)	1	Are closed system designated epidural pumps available?
	2	Is equipment standardised throughout the trust?
	3	Have medical physics been involved with identifying, checking and maintaining equipment?
	4	How will equipment malfunctions be managed?
Equipment (consumables)	1	Are appropriate consumables available e.g. 50ml leur lock syringes, non-returnable valve, type of tubing, labels for lines?

Key Factor		Associated considerations
Care of the child	1	Are there clear guidelines as to where the child will be nursed post-operatively?
	2	Is there a detailed care plan relating to pain management?
	3	Are there adequate information leaflets for the child and family?
	4	Does the care system support child and family involvement?
	5	Is there appropriate documentation?
	6	What type of monitoring and frequency of observations will be required, both during and after the infusion?
	7	Are current observation charts satisfactory? Can pain and sedation scores be recorded?
	8	How will the level of the block be assessed?
	9	How will side-effects such as respiratory depression, urinary retention, erythema and itch, nausea and vomiting, hypotension and misplaced catheters be managed?
	10	How will pressure area care be managed?
	11	Are trouble-shooting guidelines available?
	12	How will catheters be secured, wound care be managed and who will remove the catheter?
Education	1	Will there be multidisciplinary education and how will this be achieved?
	2	How will staff demonstrate competencies in care of epidural infusions?
	3	Who will assess staff and review effectiveness of educational packages?

INDEX